Stop Bingeing, *Start Living*

Proven Therapeutic Strategies for
Breaking the Binge Eating Cycle

Stop Bingeing,
Start Living

SHREIN H. BAHRAMI

ALTHEA
PRESS

Interior Designer: Christopher T. Fong
Cover Designer: Will Mack
Editor: Nana K. Twumasi
Production Editor: Andrew Yackira
Author photo © Tory Putnam

ISBN: Print 978-1-64152-100-0 | eBook 978-1-64152-101-7

R1

This book is dedicated to my clients.
Thank you for choosing me as your guide in your journey toward self-acceptance. It has been an honor and has enriched my life beyond words. And to my parents, Ahmad and Gina, thank you for your infinite love and support.

Contents

Introduction

I'm so glad you made the decision to pick up this book. Right now, you may feel low, frustrated with yourself, and unsure that change is possible. Over three million people struggle with binge eating disorder (BED), making it the most prevalent of all eating disorders. Its reach spans all genders, ages, and ethnicities. Yet the stigma, trivialization, and misinformation surrounding this mental health disorder beget secrecy and resistance toward seeking help. The consequence is evidenced by countless silent sufferers who are trapped in a deeply painful struggle far longer than they ought to be.

BED involves recurring episodes of overeating followed by intense feelings of shame—which then lead to some form of restriction in order to compensate for the binge, creating a vicious cycle. Perhaps the most harmful aspect isn't the binge itself; rather, it is the punishing and destructive self-talk followed by a desperate attempt to create a new set of unattainable dietary rules.

This reaction is not specific to BED. Anyone who suffers from any eating disorder experiences profound frustration and self-judgment regarding the inability to overcome the battle with food. However, not only do those suffering from BED ruthlessly disparage themselves, but society also reinforces the belief that their food and body problems are a result of poor self-control and a lack of willpower.

For nearly a decade, I have compassionately guided my clients to confront their fears and let go of self-limiting beliefs that have kept them stuck in a cycle of misery and hopelessness. I frequently have the honor of witnessing the transformation take place, as each individual evolves into a more authentic, grounded, and confident version of themself.

My approach to treatment is integrative and robust, drawing from evidence-based psychotherapeutic techniques as well as from the field of wellness, which addresses the mind-body-soul connection. In this book, I provide a comprehensive overview of intuitive and mindful eating philosophies, illustrating how they help build a healthier relationship with food. Within each chapter I've included questions for reflection, exercises, and specific tools for implementation.

Just as each person's history is unique, so too is their path to recovery. With that in mind, you may find parts of this book that deeply resonate with you, and others that don't. That's okay. Each chapter focuses on a facet of my approach before helping you apply what you've learned to your own unique life. When reading this book, feel free to skip exercises or sections that you're not ready to explore, and give yourself the space to move at a pace that works for you. This will help you absorb the information, process any feelings that arise, and avoid unhealthy ways of coping.

If this isn't your first attempt at healing your binge eating tendencies, try to let go of any self-criticism from earlier efforts. The most important thing is to try to remain open. The path to a healthy relationship with food is complex and varied; sometimes it takes going down several wrong paths to discover the right one, at the right time, for you. Consider how you would like this experience to be different. What might need to take a back seat in your life while you dedicate time toward your recovery? This process will start by developing clarity around why healing your relationship with food is important to you, then identifying what may be holding you back and envisioning how recovery from binge eating will impact your life. If you choose to embark on this path, I trust this book will provide you with the guidance and tools to free yourself from binge eating and enable you to step into the life you are meant to live.

CHAPTER ONE

Understanding Binge Eating

I can tell you with great assurance that it's entirely possible to break out of the torturous cycle of binge eating and the incessant mental chatter around food, your body, and self-worth. However, just as the eating disorder did not develop overnight, the changes you must make to recover will require time and patience.

In this chapter, I provide an overview of the reasons why so many people struggle to feel in control of their diet, and what typically causes someone to binge eat and develop binge eating disorder (BED). Additionally, each chapter will include anecdotes from clients I have supported in achieving recovery from BED. My intention in sharing their stories is that you might relate in some way to their experiences and realize that you are not alone. Most importantly, I hope that you believe in the possibility of your own recovery and can begin to visualize a better way of life. Next is Ruby's story; her experience is, sadly, one I hear quite often.

For the last six years, I've struggled with binge eating and have tried unsuccessfully to figure it out on my own. I've had periods of up to a few months where I don't binge, but it always returns, and I don't want to keep going on like this. I have considered getting help for so long, but I would always get sidetracked somehow. I also hate asking for help and I never knew where to start. Instead, I'd just go on another diet. It gave me the instant gratification I wanted, thinking I could fix the problem on my own with my newfound motivation. Sometimes they worked, mostly they didn't, and I always gained the weight back eventually. I am 10 pounds over my norm, and I am so tired of thinking about my food and weight 99 percent of my day. I want to control my eating so badly but feel literally incapable, like food has a spell on me. When I read the checklist for binge eating disorder, I started crying because it describes me so well. I eat in secret, I've hoarded food, I eat until I'm in physical pain, all of it. I've never been conventionally overweight, so none of my family or friends have noticed or taken it seriously. I feel exhausted trying to figure this out on my own, and I want to make a change.

When we met for our first session, Ruby was clearly overwhelmed by the constant battle in her mind about what, when, and how much to eat, as well as her deep dissatisfaction with her body. As we talked about her history with food, she recalled, as a child, frequently hiding in her closet when she felt lonely, eating handfuls of her favorite cereal directly out of the box. As a teenager, in solidarity with a few friends in preparation for prom, she went on her first diet. Since then, Ruby has been on a dieting roller coaster, trying so many diets that she's lost count. Ruby knew about anorexia and bulimia, but didn't feel that her eating problems were as acute or serious as those disorders. After reading online about binge eating, she realized she was not alone in her struggles and was ready to get the help she needed to overcome them.

Our Relationship with Food

We're born with a biological instinct to eat; our survival depends on it. Every day, we make multiple decisions as to when and what we feed ourselves. Just as no two people are exactly alike, every person has unique tastes and food preferences. Our bodies crave meal diversity and function best when receiving a balanced diet of proteins, carbohydrates, and fats. Problems arise when, instead of honoring your body's proclivities for variety and eating what you crave, you make the majority of your decisions based on what you think you *should* eat. This may involve cutting out certain foods or food groups entirely.

The idea of simplifying mealtimes by allowing only certain types of food is an attractive one, especially if it will help alleviate anxiety and reduce regret. This dilemma is addressed in the book *The Paradox of Choice*, by Barry Schwartz, which explores the impact of abundance on society. Writes Schwartz: "Freedom and autonomy are critical to our well-being, and choice is critical to freedom and autonomy. Nonetheless, though modern Americans have more choice than any group of people ever has before, and thus, presumably, more freedom and autonomy, we don't seem to be benefiting from it psychologically." People sometimes turn to diets and weight loss programs in an attempt to reduce their uneasiness around food decisions. Unfortunately, following the guidelines of a diet requires a person to not only ignore their body's cues and preferences, but to also withstand the temptation of the banned food. Inevitably, the ability to follow a diet long term becomes impossible, resulting in a binge. When this occurs, the person blames themselves for the lack of willpower and resolves to get back on the diet wagon and do it "right" the next time.

Your definition of recovery may simply be the end of bingeing. The very idea of that is most likely quite thrilling and what led you to buy this book. But it is also important to clarify what you want your relationship with food to look like. Can you envision yourself going through your day, not giving much thought to food except just before and during mealtimes? Perhaps choosing what to eat based on what your body needs, and allowing yourself to enjoy food without anxiety, judgment, or regret?

The type of relationship you have with your food usually mimics the relationship you have with yourself. How attuned are you to your needs, emotions, and desires in other areas of your life? Are you patient and flexible when the unexpected happens? Do you accept that mistakes are a part of life and move on from them? Many of my clients express wanting to find an ease and balance in their eating, yet it often becomes clear that our work together must also address creating balance in other areas of their lives.

WHY DO WE EAT WHEN WE AREN'T HUNGRY?

Our body releases chemicals—ghrelin and leptin—that signal when we need food and when we are full. Most of us frequently ignore these signals for one reason or another. Even though you might not be hungry for lunch at noon, you have a meeting at 1 p.m. and do not want to have a loud growling stomach while you share your ideas with your team. Another way we are derailed from our hunger cues is the tremendous amount of consumer marketing that is used to sell food products, brands, and experiences.

Because we all tend to label certain foods as treats, you may decide to override your level of hunger when those foods are available, like when a coworker brings in cupcakes for their birthday. Since food is so intertwined with social connections, turning down food or eating just a little of it can be perceived as rude or disrespectful.

Our emotions also trigger the urge to eat when we are not physically hungry. Here are the most common of these emotions:

Boredom: Especially for perfectionists, this feeling triggers a variety of unhealthy coping reactions. Many of my clients express feeling extremely uncomfortable with unstructured blocks of times in their day. Turning to food has become their way of filling time, as taking a break or actually relaxing may feel intolerable. It also helps to distract them from the internal voice berating them for "doing nothing."

Stress/overwhelm: Stress isn't always a bad thing, but when we allow it to build, our bodies begin to burn out from the overwhelm of holding it all in. Turning to food can be seen as a way to disconnect from the stressful thoughts and feelings by engaging the body in something seemingly comforting and generally distracting.

Loneliness: Food is a constant. It's always there and doesn't have anything negative to say. It doesn't ask you to be vulnerable or step out of your comfort zone. It's something to look forward to at the end of a long, hard day and doesn't require you to give anything in return.

Excitement: This emotion can produce a lot of energy in the body that may feel overwhelming to contain. Eating can be a way to ground the body or at least change the internal energy. Food is also something that often accompanies a celebration or event.

ENJOYING FOOD

Not only does our body send us signals indicating when we should eat, but it also releases a chemical that produces a feeling of pleasure while we eat. It is common for my clients to feel uneasy discussing the connection between food and pleasure. Pleasure in and of itself may be something they have recently/gradually become disconnected from or never felt comfortable with their entire lives. For a variety of reasons, they feel a great amount of shame acknowledging the desire for or experience of pleasure when eating and/or bingeing. Additionally, they fear that if they sanction this feeling and allow themselves to enjoy their food, the bingeing will increase and become more out of control. Yet, the result is quite the opposite. As they slow down to savor the flavors and notice how their body responds, they will feel more satisfied and content. By eating what they think will make them feel good, they choose things that are nutritious *and* tasty. Thus, the yearning that fuels mindless eating no longer exists, resulting in less over-eating and urges to binge.

Some ways to increase the enjoyment of your food and meal-times include:

- Sitting down at a table to eat, versus eating standing up, in the car/bus, or at your desk.

- Making your environment a pleasant one. For example, dim the lights, light a candle, have soft music playing, or eat outside.

- Compose your meals with a variety of colors and textures.

- Take a few deep breaths or pause for a moment of gratitude before the meal.

- Engage in mindful eating, i.e., let yourself savor each bite of food, slow your chewing, and really notice how the food feels, smells, and tastes.

- Choose foods you like, and do not force yourself to eat things you do not like the taste of.

Trusting the Process

It may feel inconceivable to even imagine having a favorable relationship with food and your body. Previous efforts may have only resulted in greater frustration and disappointment, making you want to throw up your hands and surrender. When I meet with a new client, I'm prepared for the initial caution and pessimism they may be grappling with as they seek help to end their binge eating. They often express how defeated they feel, and that, no matter how desperately ready they are to make a change, nothing they do ever seems to makes a difference. Even when they learn of others' experiences in achieving recovery, they fear they are the anomaly.

After nearly a decade of providing eating disorder treatment, I trust in the process and encourage my clients to focus not solely on the destination, but to embrace the journey as well. Your recovery may be one of the most difficult things, if not the most difficult, you face in your life. It will also be one of your greatest accomplishments. As Lao Tzu, the ancient Chinese philosopher, is often quoted as writing, "New beginnings are often disguised as painful endings." This process will in no way be pain-free. Some moments may even feel more distressing than your worst binge. Every time you face and get through these painful parts, you are closer to your new beginning. When you get there, you will look back in gratitude that you believed in yourself enough to keep going.

WHAT HAPPENS WHEN WE BINGE?

A binge typically begins with some type of provocation or trigger. These vary from person to person and occur either directly preceding the binge or up to several hours prior to the binge. Binges almost always occur in private, such as alone in a car, at home, or in the bathroom at work. Often, when one is alone, discomfort, boredom, or loneliness gives rise to a sensation of crawling out of one's skin and a very impulsive pull toward food. What follows feels like an out-of-body experience—a frantic, dissociative, or trance-like state, often occurring while standing. Binge foods tend to be ones that have been labeled as forbidden or that can't be consumed in front of others for fear of judgment. The binge episode frequently ends with extreme stomach pain and/or exhaustion.

BINGEING VARIATIONS

In addition to a variety of binge eating triggers, there are also instances where a person may regularly binge eat, but not have BED.

Night eating syndrome: This form of bingeing is characterized by an increase of food intake in the evening, and waking from sleep with the intention to eat more. Typically, this doesn't involve consuming large amounts of food, but it may occur several times in the course of a night. Even though this behavior does not always lead to weight gain, it is a common concern of those seeking help, in addition to the concurrent lack of sleep.

Sleep-related eating disorder: Those who suffer from this variation of bingeing eat while sleepwalking and are unaware of what they're doing. This is in contrast to night eating syndrome, where the individual is awake and aware of what they are eating.

You may be unsure if what you are struggling with meets the criteria for BED. It is always recommended that you consult a mental health professional in your area, but you can conduct a quick self-assessment on your own to evaluate your habits, behaviors, and emotions associated with eating.

Below are the current diagnostic criteria for a BED diagnosis, from the *Diagnostic and Statistical Manual of Mental Disorders, Fifth Edition.* As you read through the list, place check marks next to the symptoms you currently experience.

❑ You have recurrent episodes of binge eating. During these episodes, you:

- Eat an amount of food significantly larger than what a majority of people would eat in a discrete period of time

  AND

- Feel out of control during eating episodes, i.e., unable to stop eating or control how much you eat

Your episodes of binge eating are associated with three (or more) of the following:

❑ Eating more rapidly than other people would normally eat

❑ Eating until you feel uncomfortably full

❑ Eating large amounts of food when you're not feeling physically hungry

❑ Eating alone because you feel embarrassed by how much you eat

❑ Feeling disgusted with yourself, depressed, or very guilty after eating

❑ You feel distress about binge eating

❑ The binge eating occurs, on average, at least once a week for three months

❑ The binge eating is not associated with the recurrent use of inappropriate compensatory behavior (i.e., purging)

I encourage you to pause and notice any feelings you are experiencing in this moment. Do you feel similar to how Ruby felt, in that the list accurately describes your struggle? Or do only a few symptoms ring true for you? In either case, this book will help you decrease the thoughts and behaviors associated with disordered eating.

If you do not meet the requirements of the diagnostic criteria, take a moment to answer the following questions, regarding the degree to which you think about food and your body.

About how many times in a day do you

• think about your food?

• think about your body?

• compare yourself to others?

• look at/check out your body?

Are you surprised by the amount of time you spend thinking about food and your body? Has it been this way for several years, or has it changed recently? Do you have any fears around what would happen if you decrease the time you spend thinking about food and your body?

When Our Relationship with Food Goes Awry

My clients or their family will often state that a case of "healthy eating gone bad" preceded the development of an eating disorder. However, upon further discussion, they recall significant life transitions or events that occurred around the first signs of the disordered eating. Common issues that predispose someone to develop disordered eating include their childhood environment, their temperament, and cultural pressures.

OUR EVOLVING RELATIONSHIP WITH FOOD

We start out having food fed to us, and then, as we grow, our unique preferences for what we like to eat begin to take shape. Our first assertions of independence as toddlers include accepting or denying the food we are given. Yet, the environment in which we grow up significantly shapes how we relate to food. Consider your experiences with food as a child. Were mealtimes shared at the kitchen table, or was it common to eat in front of the television? Did you eat together, or was it each person for themself? Did your culture play a significant role in the type of food, quantity, or ritual aspect of family meals?

For those who grew up in a low-income household, it may not have been possible to afford fresh produce, much less organic or lean meats. Furthermore, if the providers of the family worked long hours, there may not have been time to cook, and restaurant and take-out meals might have been the norm. These factors may not feel like they're relevant to your current experience with food, but reflecting on where and how long some of the beliefs or patterns of behaviors have been around can provide clarity on why they're so hard to break.

EXERCISE   Recalling Your Family's Relationship with Food

Grab your journal and take a moment to think about how your primary caregiver(s) related to food when you were growing up. Consider the following questions, and write down your answers in as much detail as you can.

- Did your primary caregiver(s) diet or restrict certain foods?

- Did they eat different food or meals than the rest of the family?

- Did they speak positively or negatively about their weight?

- Were certain foods not present or allowed in the house?

- Did you notice differences between your household and those of other family members or friends?

- Did anyone in your family struggle with health issues like food allergies, diabetes, or other food-related problems?

Check in with yourself to see if there were any prominent feelings that arose while you read through or answered these questions. Did you make any new connections as to what may have impacted your current food issues?

It's pretty much impossible not to be impacted in some way by our primary caregiver's relationship with food. Even if their intentions were to guide you toward healthy eating habits and encourage positive body image, their own attitudes and behaviors may have led you to believe otherwise, akin to the adage, "Do as I say, not as I do." As children, we observe so much. We may ask questions, but even when we're given an honest answer, we may not understand the explanation or reasoning. We begin to form our own ways of interpreting what is good and bad, right and wrong. These interpretations can stay with us long after childhood, even in adulthood, when they are no longer logical.

THE EFFECT OF TEMPERAMENT

If our childhood environment impacts us so significantly, why is it that one sibling might develop an eating disorder while the other might not? Our temperaments are another piece of the puzzle. Temperament is defined as a person's mental, physical, and emotional traits, or one's natural predisposition. These traits are evident just weeks after birth. Were you told you were a calm and easy-going baby, or an agitated and anxious one? Your temperament impacted how you learned and expressed emotions.

You did not have access to the coping tools you now have as an adult, but food was something constant and always available to soothe, comfort, or distract. Food also may have been used as a tool to get you to behave, or as a reward—"If you clean up your room, you'll get to have ice cream for dessert!" You may associate certain foods with a loving and caring person in your life who you enjoyed being around. Do you have any affiliations with foods that are particularly soothing or comforting because of a fond childhood memory?

SOCIETY'S INFLUENCE

The effect of our societal culture on the development of disordered eating habits is profound. In 2016, Jennifer Aniston, an American actor, wrote an editorial in the *Huffington Post*, entitled "For the Record." In it, she shares her experience as a woman under the scrutiny of the paparazzi and media.

The objectification and scrutiny we put women through is absurd and disturbing. The way I am portrayed by the media is simply a reflection of how we see and portray women in general, measured against some warped standard of beauty. Sometimes cultural standards just need a different perspective so we can see them for what they really are—a collective acceptance . . . a subconscious agreement. We are in charge of our agreement. Little girls every-where are absorbing our agreement, passive or otherwise. And it begins early. The message that girls are not pretty unless they're incredibly thin, that they're not worthy of our attention unless they look like a supermodel or an actress on the cover of a magazine is something we're all willingly buying into. This conditioning is some-thing girls then carry into womanhood.

Aniston notes that our society's collective acceptance of the judgment and portrayal of women is a subconscious agreement, and that we have the power to change it if we want something different, now and for future generations. There have been steps taken by trailblazers who are ready and fighting for change now. Some examples of these initiatives are the intuitive eating approach, Health at Every Size®, and other body positive move-ments. Expect a discussion of these in chapter 4, and information on how to get involved in chapter 6.

"Quiet the mind and the soul will speak."
—Ma Jaya Sati Bhagavati, The 11 Karmic Spaces:
Choosing Freedom from the Patterns That Bind You

EXERCISE   Remembering Your History with Food

A key part of healing your relationship with food and your body is to make time for reflection. Journaling is a beneficial tool to increase insight around why your struggle with food exists and persists. As you make your way through each chapter, you will deepen your understanding of how your food beliefs developed and how they negatively impact your body image, self-esteem, and ability to listen to physical cues. In addition to completing the journaling prompts, I highly encourage you to take time to write out your thoughts and feelings during this entire process.

Now, grab your journal and take some time to write about your relationship with food as a child. Did you experience weight gain as a child or adolescent that set you on the dieting path? Were you teased or bullied because of your weight or appearance? If it is difficult to remember, you can write out some questions to ask a sibling or family member. This may help to jog your memory and process those experiences.

A SIMPLE MEDITATION

In addition to journaling, meditation allows you to connect with your thoughts and feelings in order to improve awareness and gain a sense of calmness and peace. Start in a comfortable position, ideally sitting upright with your feet on the floor. Begin by noticing the flow of your breath. Try not to judge it. Notice where your breath is originating from: your chest, stomach, or diaphragm. On your next inhale, try to gradually deepen your breath. On the inhale, count to eight, then hold your breath for two and exhale to the count of 10. Do three rounds of this. Finally, allow your breath to return to its normal state, and take note if anything changed mentally or physically.

A CULTURE OF EXCESS

Over the past few decades, the food culture in the United States has gone through significant shifts. Fast food restaurants and drive-throughs sprung up to offer families quick and inexpensive alternatives to cooking meals at home. Now, most cities have more restaurants than grocery stores, and depending on the socioeconomic status of the area, the quality and variety of fresh produce may be minimal. Buffet restaurants abound, and in general, portion sizes have grown. The standard American diet (SAD) consists of mainly red meat, dairy, processed and artificially sweetened foods, and salt, with minimal intake of fruits, vegetables, fish, and whole grains.

On the other hand, there has also been an increase in health-conscious restaurants, cafés, and grocery stores. An extreme form of this health-conscious mentality is called orthorexia. It's characterized by a hyper focus on eating healthy that becomes obsessive and provokes anxiety. It can be difficult to determine if you or someone you care about struggles with this, as orthorexic tendencies have become normalized within our culture. The distinctions for orthorexia are the degree to which a person fixates on the quality of or ingredients in their food, their ability to be flexible in different eating environments, and the level of guilt or shame they feel as a result of what they eat.

POOR HEALTH OUTCOMES

While it's okay and completely normal to overeat at times, consistent bingeing can negatively affect a person's physical and mental health. Following a binge, physical symptoms similar to a hangover can occur. This may include fatigue, listlessness, stomach pain, and gastrointestinal issues such as acid reflux. The symptoms are in response to your body working overtime, using more energy to digest the quantity of binge food. The impact on mental health, though, tends to be greater. Bingeing can send a person down a dark spiral of self-judgment, guilt, shame, and hopelessness.

If you're struggling with emotions that are inhibiting your daily functioning, reaching out to a mental health professional is imperative to feeling better. You do not have to go through this alone. See Resources on page 139 for a list of national resources for emotional and eating disorder support.

Take a few minutes to pause and reflect on your thoughts and feelings regarding the myth of "thinking thin." We'll address this myth in more detail in The Myth of "Thinking Thin" on page 20. In your journal, write out any resistance you may be feeling around letting go of the idea that thin equates to happiness. If you do not feel that you subscribe to this myth, what has contributed to that, and how do you respond to others close to you who do?

Reclaiming Your Life

A significant part of the recovery process is stepping out of the isolation that is so intertwined with binge eating. In many ways, it has inhibited you from being truly present in your life. Understandably, you may have had little interest or energy to engage in anything outside of work and life responsibilities, due to the sheer mental and physical toll of the eating disorder. As the thoughts and behaviors involved in your eating disorder begin to recede, you'll find you have more time to focus on other things, and you will physically feel stronger and more energized.

A key element for clients who have recovered has been deepening their connection with others. They began planning more activities with friends, coworkers, and family members, and held themself accountable to saying yes to invitations or not backing out at the last minute. In chapter 6, you'll learn tactics to help you navigate this shift without burning yourself out. In addition to improving your relationships, finding enjoyable activities to do with others or on your own is helpful to shift your mood and resist the urge to binge. This includes prioritizing or discovering new forms of self-care, such as reading, learning a new language, being in nature, or planning a trip.

YOU'RE NOT ALONE—
EATING DISORDER STATISTICS

Many people who struggle with an eating disorder tend to keep this struggle intensely private—enshrouded in feelings of guilt, shame, and merciless self-criticism—leading to greater isolation and division. In spite of prevention advocacy, research, and the media's attention on eating disorders, it continues to be an intensely secretive disorder. As a result, early intervention is typically rare, prolonging the recovery process and taking a toll on the sufferer's physical and mental health.

CURRENT EATING DISORDER STATISTICS AND DEMOGRAPHICS, ACCORDING TO THE NATIONAL ASSOCIATION OF ANOREXIA NERVOSA AND ASSOCIATED DISORDERS (ANAD):

- At least 30 million people of all ages and genders in the United States suffer from an eating disorder.
- Eating disorders have the highest mortality rate of any mental illness.
- From 2013 to 2016, nearly 50 percent of all American adults tried to lose weight once a year. Of those adults who tried to lose weight, 56.4 percent were women and 41.7 percent were men.
- Approximately half of one's risk for BED is genetic.
- Nearly half of those with BED have a comorbid mood disorder, such as depression or anxiety.

BREAKDOWN BY GENDER AND TYPE OF EATING DISORDER:

- .9 percent of American women and .3 percent of American men suffer from anorexia nervosa in their lifetime.
- 4 percent of American women and .5 percent of American men suffer from bulimia nervosa in their lifetime.
- 2.8 percent of American adults suffer from BED in their lifetime.

My clients have often expressed frustration or embarrassment around struggling to identify or follow through on fun activities. They are perplexed as to why it feels so hard to do things they know they will enjoy. In many ways, you must step in, just like a parent would to a child, and say to yourself, "Go outside and play!" Your days can't always be all about work and responsibilities if your goal is to live a happy and balanced life.

WHAT HAVE YOU BEEN MISSING?

This disorder has robbed you of time—time that could have been shared with people you care about or dedicated to something that supported your growth and joy. The eating disorder may have started out as an occasional respite from stressful situations, something we all deserve and need at times. But as binge eating increases, so do feelings of insecurity and anxiety around socializing. It then becomes easier to rely more on the binge eating behavior to calm nerves and feelings of isolation. Many of my clients have missed out on gatherings with friends, birthday celebrations, or vacations out of a fear of being triggered to binge or eat forbidden foods in front of others. In addition to the lost time with others, the secrecy inherent to BED can damage relationships. You may feel guilty for lying and embarrassed about possibly being seen as the "troubled one." This inhibits your ability to be intimately and authentically connected with others.

Another common thought process that causes you to miss out on satisfying life experiences is the statement, "I will do [x] when I lose weight or stop bingeing." Thinking this way keeps the exciting experiences available only in the future and only *if* you make these changes. This mentality puts life on hold and keeps you stuck not only with binge eating, but also other things in life that need to be let go. It denies you the things you want and blames the weight, when most likely it is a deep-seated feeling of unworthiness.

THE MYTH OF "THINKING THIN"

There exists a misconception that anyone can be thin as long as they try hard enough. This faulty belief system does not take into consideration the diversity of our bodies based on our genes, and our biological inability to change body shape. Do we blame people for not trying hard enough to grow taller? Further, the idea that a thin person is free from issues with food or body image is a grand fallacy. When we compare ourselves to others in this way, we rarely consider what the thin person may be struggling with, mentally or physically, and how that may be influencing their weight. Additionally, what are the costs to the quality of their lives and relationships if they are manipulating their hunger and body to maintain a low weight?

Imagine two thin women who have very similar diets and exercise regimens. One feels great about her body and food choices, spending zero to minimal time questioning meal decisions or feeling guilty that she could have fit in more time at the gym. The other woman believes that there is always room for improvement and continually wishes for more self-control around food choices and portions. She berates herself for not working out hard enough and constantly compares her routine to others. Their dichotomous perceptions about themselves and feelings differ greatly, even though their weight is the same. Further, the woman who judges herself is more likely to engage in self-sabotage and retaliatory behaviors such as making impulsive food choices or bingeing.

LEARNING TO EAT SUSTAINABLY

Healing your disordered eating means reframing your relationship with food and learning to listen to your body. This approach involves little discussion on *what* you should be eating and instead focuses more on the *why*. When you allow yourself to eat whatever you want, without guilt or judgment, the biological and mental urges to binge will begin to diminish. Your body is not a robot or machine. Hunger cues and taste preferences change constantly. As long as you stay attuned to the cues and feed yourself regularly, your body will feel satiated and trust that it will be fed again. No longer will your survival instincts be triggered due to deprivation or meal inconsistency.

Getting the Most out of This Book

The following chapters dive into what it takes to end binge eating. Chapters 2 and 3 explain the most current, evidence-based approaches to healing binge eating and how you can set manageable goals in applying these techniques to your own recovery. I encourage you to go at your own pace, but I also recommend putting some accountability in place now to help you stay on track. Carving out blocks of time in your schedule to continue reading, journaling, and sharing your process with someone supportive will help keep you motivated and closer to your goals.

Chapter 4 suggests ways in which you can become better connected to your body's cues and provides some practical nutrition education. In chapter 5, you'll explore your range of emotion and discover how you can experience feelings without causing emotional eating. In chapter 6, you'll be given concrete tools to apply these steps in your daily life.

CHAPTER TWO

Packing Your Toolkit

Disordered eating is a learned behavior that can be replaced over time. Your brain has the capacity to change by forming new connections when you consistently engage in healthier, more productive, or more enjoyable activities. In order to make these new activities stick, there must be a clear understanding as to why the binge behaviors began and how they have served you in your life. It may feel odd to consider that the BED behaviors are in any way efficacious, but they would not have formed if they did not serve a purpose and were not positively reinforced.

Katie is a client who reached out after making changes in several areas in her life that caused her significant distress. In spite of the emotional toll, she was feeling inspired to address the greatest factor in her unhappiness: her weight.

> *Over the last several years, I have gone through some major life transitions. I divorced my husband of 10 years, moved out of our home, and am living alone for the first time in my life. I also left my job in tech after earning my MBA, and started my own nonprofit business supporting women in impoverished countries. After navigating my divorce and career change, I am a total believer that if I put my mind toward something,*

and am open to support from others, I can accomplish it. During the process of getting divorced, I read several books on the topic and even joined a divorce support group. These things helped me tremendously—I no longer feel so alone and ostracized from my friends who are married. I slowly stopped beating myself up so much for the failure of my marriage. Now, I want to apply these changes in my life to end my binge eating. I have been overweight my whole life. I feel so frustrated that I really have no idea how to eat normally, and I fear it is too late for me. Growing up, I watched my mom measure her food and track her calories; eventually, I did the same. I honestly think I have read every diet book out there! My biggest weight loss was for my wedding, when I basically cut my daily calories in half. Not only did I eventually regain all the weight back, but since then I've been at the highest weight I've ever been and fear that I've done irreparable damage to my metabolism. On top of the weight cycling, I realize now that doing those things just makes me more paranoid and focused on my food, not more in control of it. I've been reading about the benefits of mindfulness and how dieting does not work, but I am terrified of letting go of a lifetime of dieting because there is still a part of me that thinks I can get it right with the next diet.

When we started our work together, Katie was aware that partaking in the continuous cycle of dieting had ultimately left her feeling profoundly disconnected from her body. In order to create a more attuned and respectful relationship with her body, she would need to learn how to change her diet mind-set and address old belief systems.

EXERCISE   Basic Mindful Eating Activity

Eating mindfully means paying conscious attention to the experience of eating. It involves eating while noticing and attuning to all five senses, without judgment, with moment-to-moment awareness, and noting the range of flavors and textures within each bite. By engaging in mindful eating, you can gain clarity around your thoughts and feelings toward food.

For most people with BED, this is a radically new approach to eating, and you will likely experience some degree of resistance to slowing down and being truly present with your food. Dieting teaches us that food is the enemy and must be dispensed with quickly. The reality is that food and eating are central to life. Eating mindfully at every meal and snack, while uncomfortable and perhaps awkward at first, is entirely possible and is an important first step to changing your relationship with food. Beginning a mindfulness practice, no matter how small, can be immensely helpful in healing disordered eating, as well as helping in other areas of your life.

For this activity, you may begin by simply choosing one piece of food—such as a piece of chocolate, a raisin, a slice of watermelon— or a complete meal.

1 Create a relaxing ambiance by putting on quiet or soothing music, lighting a candle, or dimming the lights.

2 Become aware of your hunger level.

3 Sit down at a table.

4 Note the smell, texture, and temperature of your food.

5 Take the time to chew. Try for at least 10 chews per bite, and note whether you prefer to chew on one side of your mouth or the other. Pause to take a drink, and notice the qualities of what you are sipping (is it cold, warm, bubbly, refreshing?).

6 Put your utensils down while you chew.

7 Periodically notice your hunger level until you end your meal.

After eating, think or journal about the emotions you felt during the exercise. Was it a pleasant or unpleasant experience? Are you looking forward to eating in this manner again? Consider your thought habits. Were you critiquing your food choice or manner of eating? As you note these thoughts, try to label them: self-criticism, guilt, pleasure, frustration, etc. Remember, there is no right or wrong answer here. This is an exercise to bring your attention to the experience of eating, and, like any newly acquired skill, it takes practice and repetition.

"Between stimulus and response there is a space.
In that space is our power to choose our response.
In our response lies our growth and our freedom."
—*Unknown*

Eating Mindfully and Intuitively

By transitioning to mindful and intuitive eating, you will begin to alter or end long-standing habits that have contributed to your binge eating. Mindful eating has to do with *how* you eat, while intuitive eating is about listening to the innate wisdom of your body. These practices will redevelop your ability to notice the cues that have long been overruled by the diet guidelines. Those cues exist because the organism that is our physical body signals us to eat *what we need*. While it is anathema to the falsehoods that come from the billion-dollar diet industry, the truth is that our bodies encourage us to eat in ways that will sustain us and bring us to health.

Mindful and intuitive eating help us learn to trust our bodies to lead us to appropriate nourishment. When we are attuned to our bodies, we make food choices that will satisfy our needs and quiet the mental churn of diet rules that lead us to question every food choice.

MINDFUL EATING

Statistics show that people consume more food when they multitask at mealtimes. Are you someone who must have a book or magazine with you when you eat? Or do you typically eat in front of a TV or laptop? These are all methods of disconnection and distraction. By not being present and focused on the act of eating, you lose the ability to tune into your body's signals, and this disconnect can lead you to overeat.

According to The Center for Mindful Eating, someone who eats mindfully:

- acknowledges that there is no right or wrong way to eat, only varying degrees of awareness surrounding the experience of food

- accepts that their eating experiences are unique

- directs their awareness to all aspects of food and eating on a moment-by-moment basis

- focuses on the immediate choices and direct experiences associated with food and eating, not on the distant health outcome of those choices

- is aware of and reflects on the effects of unmindful eating

- reflects on how they can act to achieve specific health goals as they become more attuned to the direct experience of eating and feelings of health

- is aware of the interconnection of the Earth, living beings, and cultural practices, and the impact of their food choices on those systems

The first step to eating more mindfully is to notice the initial desire to eat, then pause and ask yourself why you want to eat. Is it because of a feeling (i.e., anger, joy, boredom), a form of habit (i.e., same time of day), or does your body need the fuel? In other words, is the cue to eat a result of a desire to meet an emotional need, or is your body telling you it needs nourishment? Either reason is valid, but understanding the "why" helps you become more aware of your needs and better prepares you to craft a just right response. That "just right response" can be to fill a need for nourishment, but it can also be because eating is the best option you have for caring for yourself at that particular moment. Being conscious of why you are choosing to eat puts you in a position of strength. As a result, you are choosing your method of self-care, and eating isn't happening to you in an out-of-control way.

For example, let's say you had a particularly rough day, and you arrive home after work tired and cold. You dash in the door and sit down with a cup of hot cocoa and a cookie as a way of addressing the unpleasant feelings and comforting your mind and body. While sitting with the warm mug in your hand, you pause to think about why it was such a rough day. You recall how the day began with a strongly worded email from your boss that shifted your mood immediately. For the rest of the day, you felt on edge and were short with your colleague when telling her you didn't have time to go on your regular 20-minute walk together during lunch. With this clarity, you set an intention of repairing things with your colleague and committing to the afternoon walk the next day.

The alternative scenario, the one where mindfulness and attunement are absent, may look like the following: Ignoring your feelings, you walk in the door and force yourself to do more work in order to get ahead for the next day. At some point, you look up from your computer and realize it's late and you haven't eaten. You feel physically and mentally exhausted, with no clarity of mind to make food decisions that are responsive to your needs. You choose whatever is easiest and decide to make a bowl of cereal. Yet, on so many levels that feels unsatisfying. Your frustration and disconnect grow, so you pour yourself another bowl . . . and then another. While you're trying desperately to meet a need, the method isn't helping because you don't know what need you're trying to fix. Continuing to eat the cereal takes you farther away from accurate or specific self-care and elicits misery, guilt, and frustration. You wake up the next morning with no resolution around your feelings and an added layer of binge regret.

INTUITIVE EATING

The intuitive eating philosophy was developed by registered dietitians Evelyn Tribole and Elyse Resch in 1995. Their approach came about from providing nutritional counseling to clients, suffering through their own personal struggles with food, and witnessing the detrimental effects and futile efforts of dieting. After years of treating clients, Tribole and Resch saw the diet industry for what it was: a hugely successful moneymaking business that capitalizes on people feeling like failures and becoming repeat customers. Dieters beat themselves up for "failing yet again" and—inevitably—search for the next diet plan that will finally do the trick. Tribole and Resch came to realize that switching the focus to lifestyle changes and learning to follow one's own internal guide created the greatest amount of positive change in a person's diet and overall health.

As I mentioned in chapter 1, we were born with the innate ability to know when we need to eat, how much, and even what type of food we need at a given time. However, we've been told for a number of reasons that we cannot trust our bodies and should strive to overcome and triumph over our biological needs. Clients tell me, in great frustration, "I don't know how to eat anymore, I have no idea what my body wants." Our survival mechanisms (that have allowed our species to evolve and thrive) will respond when restricted or deprived of food options and manifest odd behaviors in order to meet our bodies' needs. Becoming attuned to your body, allowing yourself to eat within an all-foods-fit framework, free from beliefs regarding right/wrong or good/bad, initiates the process of rebuilding trust and returning to your body's intuitive wisdom.

This is not to say that if your body wants three candy bars every day, you should follow its plea and call this intuitive eating. A component of your recovery may mean allowing yourself those candy bars, scary as it may sound, in order to learn that eating candy bars is acceptable if you have determined that candy bars are truly what you need/want on a given day. When foods are allowed to leave the arbitrary judgment categories of good/bad, they lose the power to be binge foods. Instead, they become just one of a myriad of food options. Identifying and understanding why a part of you wants the candy bar will help you make the right decision (for you) and short-circuit the automatic pathway to guilt and misery.

Understanding Every "Part" of Yourself

The concept of having different parts of yourself may be new to you, but we all experience dialogues in our mind regarding a variety of things. Typically, thoughts tend to be around either what needs to get done or issues from the past. The way we perceive and process life experiences has a tremendous impact on our mood. When you notice a shift in your mood, it may be because your perspective has shifted or a different part of you has stepped in.

Say it's your birthday and you wake up feeling excited and happy. After getting dressed, your mood goes south, as you do not like how you look in the outfit you chose. You change clothes, but only feel more uncomfortable throughout the day, and your mood continues to sink until you return home from work. You decide to not let the bad mood ruin your evening, and rally yourself to enjoy the celebratory dinner your friends prepared for you. In each of the different moods experienced throughout the day, there was a

KEY PRINCIPLES OF INTUITIVE EATING

Tribole and Resch compiled a list of 10 key principles in their book, *Intuitive Eating: A Revolutionary Program that Works.*

1. **Reject the diet mentality:** The diet mentality is the idea that there's a diet out there somewhere that will work for you. Intuitive eating is the anti-diet.

2. **Honor your hunger:** Hunger is not your enemy. Respond to your early signs of hunger by feeding your body. If you let yourself get excessively hungry, you are likely to overeat.

3. **Make peace with food:** Call a truce in the war with food. Get rid of ideas about what you should or shouldn't eat.

4. **Challenge the food police:** Food is not good or bad, and you are not good or bad for what you eat or don't eat. Challenge thoughts that tell you otherwise.

5. **Respect your fullness:** Just as your body tells you when it is hungry, it also tells you when it is full. Listen for the signals of comfortable fullness, when you feel you've had enough. As you're eating, check in with yourself to see how the food is tasting and how hungry or full you are feeling.

6. **Discover the satisfaction factor:** Make your eating experience enjoyable. Have a meal that tastes good to you. Sit down to eat it. When you make eating a pleasurable experience, you might find it takes less food to satisfy you.

7. **Honor your feelings without using food:** Emotional eating is a strategy for coping with feelings. Find other ways that are not related to food to deal with your feelings: take a walk, meditate, journal, call a friend. Become aware of the times when a feeling that you might call hunger is actually based in emotion.

8. **Respect your body:** Rather than criticizing your body for how it looks and what you perceive is wrong with it, recognize it as capable and beautiful, just as it is.

9. **Exercise—feel the difference:** Find ways to move your body that you enjoy. Shift the focus from losing weight to feeling energized, strong, and alive.

10. **Honor your health—gentle nutrition:** The food you eat should taste good and feel good. Remember that it's your overall food patterns that shape your health. One meal or snack isn't going to make or break your health.

part of you chiming in, directing your thoughts and feelings. All parts have a vested interest in how you live your life.

When my clients are learning to eat more mindfully, I will often encourage them to name a part of themselves that will take on the role of the nurturing and authoritative parent. Especially in the beginning phases of intuitive eating, bringing a perspective of curiosity and patience in order to understand the situation, weigh the pros and cons, and make an informed decision will make all the difference. This is in direct contrast to the other parenting styles: authoritarian (the diet mentality, comprised of total rigidity akin to a dictatorship), permissive (the binge mentality, comprised of anarchy that feels like a chaotic free-for-all), or negligent (a subhead of the binge mentality, comprised of absolute disregard and neglectfulness). When you question what part of you wants that third brownie, it is like being the parent who gently and lovingly guides their child to discover *for themselves* what is best for them.

Consider the part of you that impacts your relationship with food. If that part of you is a younger version of yourself, what does it really need? If it's your rebellious side and it's saying, "Screw my boss! I'm eating this whole gallon of ice cream," can you listen to that part of you? Can you be the nurturing parent who helps identify what the underlying feelings are, and soothe, comfort, and care for that need? The alternative is to temporarily respond to the part by angrily eating the gallon of ice cream or "checking out" altogether with mindless eating, only to later feel miserable and stuck once again.

LETTING GO OF UNFRIENDLY VALUES

You may apply certain values to food that go against your true physical hunger. I call these "unfriendly" values. For example, you may tell yourself you must finish everything on your plate at a restaurant because you paid for it, or because throwing food away is like throwing money down the drain. So, you eat everything in accordance with that value, rather than mindfully tuning in to determine how full you are. Another instance might occur at an event or party where there is a plethora of free food. You think, "It's free food, I have to take advantage of it!" or "When will I get to eat this particular dish again? I better have as much as I can." Adhering to unfriendly values can take you far away from listening to the innate wisdom of your body. To be clear, there is nothing wrong with enjoying some delicious food provided at a party or delighting in a second slice of pie simply because it tastes so darn good, so long as you are honoring your body and not disregarding it by checking out, stuffing it to discomfort, or blindly following these unfriendly values.

> "When we give up dieting, we take back something we were often too young to know we had given away: our own voice. Our ability to make decisions about what to eat and when. Our belief in ourselves. Our right to decide what goes into our mouths. Unlike the diets that appear monthly in magazines or the thermal pants that sweat off pounds, unlike a lover or a friend or a car, your body is reliable. It doesn't go away, get lost, stolen. If you will listen, it will speak."
> —Geneen Roth, Breaking Free from Emotional Eating

Striving Beyond Weight Loss

The greatest reason for not following your own internal eating compass tends to be the desire to lose weight. If weight loss is your ultimate goal, it forces you to focus not on what your body needs, but what will bring about a decrease in the number on the scale. If you've been a chronic dieter, both your body and mind will need time and continued practice to acclimate to a more mindful approach. It may be terrifying to trust that the lack of rules and structure will result in a better, healthier life. Diet plans claim to provide you with a direct road to weight loss and happiness. The idea of eating when hungry and stopping when full seems far too precarious. Being an intuitive eater does not mean that the urge to eat when not physically hungry will disappear, it just means that you will become aware of emotional and physical hunger and therefore be able to respond mindfully to those cues.

Perhaps you're having a lovely time at a friend's birthday party and decide you would like to eat a piece of cake just like everyone else. That's terrific, because you're aware that you want to celebrate with food even if your stomach isn't grumbling for lack of sustenance. To be an intuitive and mindful eater, you must make the choice to prioritize physical and mental health over losing weight. This is not giving up; this is your way out of the cycle of deprivation that does not deliver on what it promises.

DEMYSTIFYING THE MYTH OF WILLPOWER

Diet experts have extolled the belief that willpower is the determining factor in a person's ability to follow a diet. For those who eat intuitively, food holds no power. Intuitive eaters' bodies operate in an optimal range of energy because they respond to hunger cues that indicate when and what to eat. When their energy level begins to dip, the body sends a signal to be refueled. And when given the amount of food needed, the person feels satiated and energized.

Thus, the false concept of "just needing willpower" in order to eat well is rendered moot. There's no need for a storm of negative and relentless thoughts about calories, choices about eating/not eating, good/bad food comparisons, body size shaming, guilt, or punishment. Instead, the body has what it needs, and the mind and heart are free to fully participate in life.

PUSHING PAST RESISTANCE

Mindful and intuitive eating fly right in the face of everything advocated by the diet industry. When I introduce these philosophies to clients, they understandably experience some anxiety and skepticism. These approaches are inherently saying *they* must pick up the reins and discover what is right for *them*. In order to end their bingeing and feel in control of their food, they must listen to and restore trust with their bodies. An initial response I typically hear is, "Can I lose some weight first, and *then* commit to eating intuitively?" This is essentially asking to have both approaches: Let go of the eating disorder and finally feel freedom, while also holding on to the old methods in case this radical new way doesn't work. Yet, if an eating disorder specialist colludes with the eating disorders' absolute demand for rules and rigidity, we let our clients down.

I don't expect that my clients will simply stop wanting to lose weight, but it cannot *just* be about weight loss. Unlike diets or working with a weight loss coach, our work together is focused on ending the unhealthy eating behaviors and establishing goals that support clients' health, well-being, and quality of life. Success is not measured by numbers on a scale or the amount of willpower my clients demonstrate; rather, it is about being in sync with one's body, mind, needs, and desires.

FACING YOUR FEARS

Your decision to read this book may have been driven by a desire to decrease the amount of time you spend thinking about food. You may feel that you are already mindful about your eating and want to learn how to focus your mind on more important things. The idea of increasing your awareness around your thoughts, feelings, and body may feel overwhelming. I get it and agree; you deserve a break! However, what I am proposing actually differs

ON MINDFULNESS

It may be unclear what mindfulness is exactly. Some confuse it with meditation and think it means sitting in a cross-legged position on a pillow for an hour. What mindfulness really encourages us to do is to get off autopilot. Mindfulness allows us to create pauses in our day and notice what is taking place in that moment, without judgment or thoughts of the past or future. The idea behind mindfulness is to take every experience as it is, look at it from different angles, and remain open to new possibilities. Our minds will instinctively want to categorize our experiences by referencing the past, and by lumping things together to file away as further proof and evidence of our beliefs. We must pause and dismantle the assumption that our thoughts are facts.

There is no right or wrong way to practice mindfulness. By simply pausing and noticing your breath, you are being mindful. If, while driving, you pause to think about the current moment instead of where you are going, whether you will be late, or if you'll be able to find parking once you arrive, you are being mindful. It is a way of helping you stay present with what is going on around you and create the space to allow you to choose an action that is aligned with your values and goals. You can also begin to see more clearly the habits that you would like to change. Mindfulness can be an instrumental tool in ending bingeing and living the life you want.

from the ways you may have been ruminating on your relationship with eating.

A common fear expressed by my clients is that an increased focus on food will trigger even more binge eating. Just the idea of giving themselves permission to enjoy food and eat what they want conjures visions of gorging on food and never being able to stop. But the reality is you're feeling out of control with food now, in spite of all the rules. Food and hunger are not the enemy; you are not the enemy. The damage has come from forcing our exquisitely designed body to operate by some arbitrary system that demands us to disconnect our physical and emotional selves when we eat.

The approach I suggest actually returns control (or more precisely said, restores harmony) in our relationships with hunger, satiety, and food. If, as you start out, you find you have "lost control" during one of the many times you will be eating, simply note it and seek to understand what was happening at that particular time. Awareness yields data that is useful for the next time you eat.

My clients also fear that they won't be able to manage the intense self-judgment that might arise if they find pleasure in food. This fear is valid and, for many, will be a meaningful part of the work in learning this new approach. As you make your way through this book, you will learn ways to eat mindfully, even if the critical voice in your head is having a major tantrum. One of the many amazing things I get to witness as I travel this journey with my clients is their ability to quiet and better manage the critical voices (or what I sometimes refer to as the "mean committee") in their heads. It may not seem like it now, but it's entirely possible to develop a new relationship with yourself. As you challenge yourself in ways you never thought possible, you will begin to feel the shift within, and sense the connection to your internal source of power and self-trust.

EXERCISE   Activity for Addressing Cravings or Urges

A strategy I frequently suggest to help clients override urges to binge is called opposite action. It is from a treatment approach called Dialectical Behavior Therapy, which was developed in the late 1980s by psychologist Marsha M. Linehan. This approach integrates mindfulness and cognitive behavioral therapy to help people better regulate their emotions and improve their interpersonal skills. Specifically, the opposite action strategy has been used effectively to help people who suffer from disordered eating. Follow these steps to use opposite action when you feel the urge to binge:

1   Identify the emotion(s) you are experiencing.

2   Determine whether the emotion and its intensity are appropriate for the present situation.

3   Decide whether acting on the urge will be in your best interests, in line with your values, or effective in the long term.

4   Either act on the urge or choose an act that is opposite to the urge.

When you follow these steps, you are not ignoring, negating, or avoiding your emotions. Instead, this strategy helps put you in the driver's seat to decide on the appropriate response. For example, if you are experiencing feelings of worthlessness, the urge may be to do something self-destructive. The opposite would be to engage in self-care or give care to someone else. Or, if you're feeling angry, the urge may be to yell and throw something. The opposite action would be to speak in a composed manner or not respond at all. By choosing the opposite action, you improve your ability to stabilize your mood, avoiding the downward emotional spiral that used to trigger a binge. Being able to regulate your emotions will allow you to make the right call and will get you to a more equitable emotional state.

Rewiring Your Brain

A healthy relationship with food also includes how we think and feel about ourselves. One of the most scientifically tested and highly effective psychotherapeutic approaches is cognitive behavioral therapy (CBT). This approach helps us understand why we behave the way we do, and offers a wealth of strategies for rerouting the negative ways we think and feel about ourselves. It is a structured, present-oriented treatment approach that focuses on changing flawed thought patterns that create harmful habits and behaviors.

HOW CBT WORKS

CBT uses a variety of techniques to help people improve not only the decisions they make, but also their overall quality of life. Since its premise is based on the idea that how a person *perceives* a situation informs their reaction more than the situation itself, the treatment's focus must center on what impacts one's perception. This is done through a number of thought and belief tracking exercises. Again, similar to mindfulness approaches, when we shine a light on why we think the way we do, we create the opportunity to alter our thinking.

WHY CBT WORKS TO HEAL BINGE EATING

CBT can be used to heal disordered eating in a number of ways. First, many of the disordered or obsessive actions around food are due to strongly held beliefs, like *being thin equates to happiness*. Second, those who struggle with food or body issues often compare themselves to others and presume that their issues are a result of a lacking in willpower they believe others possess. As a result of this perception, self-critical beliefs are reinforced or created, cementing fears of being different, broken, or that recovery is just not in the cards for them.

In her book, *Big Girl*, Kelsey Miller powerfully addresses this misconception: "We call fat people lazy. They're not. Fat people are zealous. They will cleave and push and fight harder than anyone. They have been in battle since the day someone poked them in the soft part of their belly or slapped the last piece of Halloween candy from their chubby hand. No one works harder at anything than a fat person works on a diet they believe will make them thin."

This experience is congruous to my client Katie's, whose story I shared at the beginning of this chapter. She felt embittered by the fact that she could be successful in her career, yet her issues with food and her weight seemed insurmountable. The belief that she simply did not have enough willpower did not add up. How could she have made it through her divorce, earned a master's degree, and started her own business without a tremendous amount of self-discipline and strength?

I am consistently impressed by my clients' achievements and levels of intelligence. Yet, they remain stuck in their disordered eating despite countless attempts to change. This is because the problem is not a battle of wills, but about who holds the power. The reason why some people can live a life free of food issues is that food holds no power over them. When you make food choices out of fear, an internal conflict is created as your body fights to get its needs met and maintain homeostasis. It will do this in several ways, including slowing or increasing the metabolism and producing intense hunger cues and cravings.

DISTORTIONS OF THE MIND

One way you can tackle negative thought patterns is to consider if they are cognitive distortions, or ways the mind convinces you of something that isn't true. Just a few of the most common cognitive distortions are listed next. As you read through, try to recall a time you experienced thinking in this way.

All-or-Nothing (Black-and-White) Thinking: This is a desire to assign something as good or bad. When my clients use the words *should*, *always*, or *never*, I ask if they are stuck in this distortion and if, by taking a step back, they could find the grey area. An example of this would be eating intuitively the entire day, but then feeling uncomfortably full after eating dessert and therefore classifying the day as a failure. Instead, reflecting on the wins and struggles is a more fair and balanced way of assessing your recovery progress.

Overgeneralization: This way of thinking is like a downward spiral into a black hole, where a single negative event is used as proof that everything else will go wrong, too. An example would be getting a "C" on a test, and then dropping the class because you believe you will never be able to pass it.

Jumping to Conclusions: Also known as mind reading or fortune-telling, this is when someone assumes they know what other people think about them—usually projected as something negative—and believes it as fact. An example would be meeting your coworkers for the first time and assuming they are all thinking, "How did *he* get this job?"

Mental Filter: Mental filtering occurs when you recall a situation and only focus on the negative aspects, filtering out anything positive. An example would be if a friend comes to visit your new home, and though they make an abundance of compliments, their one negative comment is the only thing you remember.

Personalization: This is when a person places all of the responsibility or blame on their own shoulders, causing unreasonably high amounts of guilt and regret. An example would be if you are hosting a party and a friend of yours gets into a fender bender on the way to your house. Personalization would have you blame yourself for the accident, since it happened on the way to your party.

REWIRING THE URGE TO BINGE

One of the most difficult challenges of healing BED is navigating the moments preceding a binge. The urge to binge typically involves a combination of thoughts and physical sensations that cause great discomfort. Habitual patterns are formed when it feels like the only way to end the intolerable feeling is to do the behavior. In the book, *You Are Not Your Brain*, Jeffrey Schwartz applies CBT principles to help you uncross the wires that lead to habitual problematic behaviors:

Step 1—Name It: Become more conscious of your thoughts and emotions by identifying and naming them.

Step 2—Frame and Function: Take a step back and try to recognize the trigger to the thoughts and feelings. Determine what you think the purpose of the trigger is; what is it truly needing/wanting?

Step 3—See Yourself: To begin to rewire your brain, imagine yourself not giving in to a binge. Visualize yourself ignoring the urge to binge and doing something more fulfilling and beneficial to your health and happiness instead. Really paint a picture of this in your mind, as the power of visualization is incredibly effective for actualizing our intentions.

Step 4—Focus: Each time you have an urge to binge, redirect your thoughts to something that is very important to you. Think of someone you care about or a project or cause you feel passionate about. In this step, you are actually rewiring your brain. The more times you go through these steps as you experience an urge, the less powerful the urge becomes.

Now it's your turn to consider your perception of things, the thoughts that form as a result, and their impact on your behaviors. This does not have to be complicated. Whenever you engage in an undesired behavior (related to food or not), make a note of what you think the preceding thought(s) were. Secondly, determine if any of your thoughts fit one of the cognitive distortions presented on page 40.

Accept and Commit

Another approach that has been empirically shown to support recovery in people with disordered eating is acceptance and commitment therapy (ACT). Just like the acronym suggests, this method involves taking action in order to change or recover. By taking action, as opposed to solely talking through your fears, you are able to more effectively challenge the fears and anxiety that have been holding you back. Most likely, these deeply rooted fears and anxiety began during childhood. As children, we have very few options to address our emotional pain. In order to get through discomfort when we were younger, we avoided it, acted out, or blamed ourselves and tried to fix it in some way.

To heal these damaging thoughts and behaviors, you must be willing to name the feelings you've avoided and experience them. This could mean reflecting and writing about them in a journal or a voice or video recording; or talking to someone supportive, such as a close friend or therapist. The second step is to allow the feelings to just be, rather than judging, dismissing, or jumping to fix them. As you do so, trust that they will not last forever, and accept them as they are. Unlike many external things in your life, these feelings cannot be controlled. When you stop trying to control or avoid feelings, the internal conflict that keeps you from moving through an emotion will subside.

IDENTIFYING YOUR VALUES

The ACT approach operates on the belief that naming your values will keep you dedicated to the hard work necessary to recover. Integrating your values into your life now, rather than in later stages of recovery, will cement the critical lifestyle changes necessary to end disordered eating. Taking time to assess and reevaluate your values will help you shift your focus away from food and toward the things that truly matter. Contrary to goals, values are not things that can be accomplished or mastered. For example, the value of being a good friend cannot be accomplished in a finite way. Values require consistent and ongoing attention, and are upheld through practices that support them over time, rather than a singular act or achievement. We will talk more about values in chapter 3.

ACCEPTING THE OUTCOMES

One of the major components of the ACT approach is accepting your thoughts and feelings and acknowledging that you cannot control or run from them. Instead, you are encouraged to observe them without judgment. This means that by accepting your feelings, you accept *all* feelings, which will include suffering of some kind. The belief that life can be lived without suffering is false and creates *more* suffering as you try to reach this unattainable destination.

Understanding and accepting suffering is a key component of Buddhist teachings. Sharon Salzberg, an author and a leading figure in the field of meditation and modern Buddhist teaching, puts it in simple terms in her book, *A Heart as Wide as the World*: "This denial of suffering often occurs in family life. Sometimes there is great suffering in a family—discord, conflict, insecurity, violence—and in an effort to shield children from the truth, a great silence descends: the silence of denial, and of avoidance. If it is ever talked about, the suffering is repackaged and manipulated to look like something else."

Because the resistance to suffering is often learned at a very young age, it can be a difficult mentality to break free from, leading many people to cope with unhealthy methods like eating disorders. By breaking this cycle, you create a new family legacy in which to navigate emotions and conflict.

The ACT approach considers our strong desire for control and addresses how important it is to recognize what actually is and is not within our control. By understanding that, as human beings, we all suffer, have flaws, and make mistakes, we can engage in actively accepting these aspects of our human nature.

COMMITTING TO THE PROCESS

In order to truly make progress in your recovery and end your binge eating behaviors, you must be willing to make a commitment to yourself and to the process. To do this, it is important to recognize what barriers may keep you from following through, and what could take you off course. When I ask clients, "What could get in the way of your recovery?" their response is almost always, "Myself." But what does that mean exactly? When I ask for more details, the list often includes time, work, life responsibilities, family expectations, other health concerns, social pressure, and finances. These are all very important considerations that cannot be disregarded or simply cut out. But, with intention, space can be made for your recovery work.

> "What you're supposed to do when you don't
> like a thing is change it. If you can't change
> it, change the way you think about it."
> —Maya Angelou, Wouldn't Take Nothing
> for My Journey Now

ADDING TO YOUR RECOVERY TOOLBOX

Acceptance and commitment therapy (ACT) and cognitive behavioral therapy (CBT) are research-based techniques that have been used in the treatment of mental health issues for years. Two of the more recent approaches for healing disordered eating (as well as improving mindfulness, contentment, and peace of mind) include:

Self-Compassion: This is an approach developed by Dr. Kristin Neff that addresses the significance of accepting and honoring our own humanity and decreasing the amount of self-criticism and judgment we constantly flood ourselves with. You may try to change in ways that allow you to be healthier and happier, but this is done because you care about yourself, not because you're worthless or unacceptable as you are. If you solely use self-criticism as motivation, it will make you lose faith in yourself. Here are the three elements of self-compassion:

- Self-kindness vs. self-judgment
- Common humanity vs. isolation
- Mindfulness vs. over-identification

Radical Acceptance: This approach, by Tara Brach, PhD, addresses the significance of being able to surrender to the things in life that are out of your control by accepting them as reality. This frees you from the suffering that would typically ensue if you fought against the truth. By acknowledging what has taken place, you are better able to use the feelings that arise as information on how to respond. This may mean changing how you verbally or behaviorally respond in the moment or when the situation occurs again. Conversely, when we become indignant or attached to a certain outcome of what we think should happen, we react (typically in a negative, destructive way). For many who struggle with disordered eating, this philosophy of acceptance is also crucial to addressing weight and body image concerns.

Make two columns in your journal: one titled "Reasons to Keep My Eating Disorder" and the other titled "Reasons to Let Go of My Eating Disorder." Take your time adding items to each, reflecting on how recovery will truly change your life, and what it may bring about or take away. Include barriers that have gotten in the way in the past, and consider what could come up for you in the following weeks and months.

Next Steps

Now that you've learned some of the most widely used approaches for treating disordered eating, I'll address ways that you can keep yourself accountable and motivated while applying these strategies to your day-to-day life. You'll discover what might still be holding you back from recovery, and what will make this journey worth it. We'll also assess what you value in life and what you hope to create in the future.

CHAPTER THREE

Your Goals and Values

This chapter focuses on how you can successfully adopt the strategies that will enable you to bring an end to your disordered eating. In my initial consultation with clients, they often express how much time and effort they have already invested in improving their knowledge around nutrition. Yet, in spite of the tremendous amount of education, their eating disorder continues to persist. Sara, age 45, reached out to me as she was struggling to stay on track with her eating disorder recovery. She felt that she had done a lot of work so far, yet the tools were just not clicking for her:

> *I truly think that I am obsessed with or addicted to food. I hear myself talking about my weight nonstop; it occupies 99 percent of my daily thoughts. I'm sick of feeling like I constantly fail at eating, never having enough willpower to ignore the urges to binge. I want to feel more comfortable in my clothes and fit into things in my closet that I haven't worn in years. I want to feel truly confident in myself, not just in my work. I'm tired of never feeling good enough and how my weight completely determines my self-worth. I want more*

*energy, and to be more positive. I want to feel like I'm moving forward
in health and weight loss goals—not stuck. I want to find the spark
of motivation that I can hold on to. I do a lot of research. I feel like I
already know the answers to my problems. Sometimes I feel like I have
control and I am eating well and very active, but I always seem to find
myself eventually back in a cycle like this. I am worried that I am the
exception to the rule and will never recover.*

Just like Katie in chapter 2, Sara had a very successful career.
To those around her, she appeared to be doing very well in
life. She kept her struggles with food secret from her husband
and closest friends, fearing the roadblocks she kept coming up
against were intimations of something inherently wrong with her.
She struggled to understand why she couldn't handle, or didn't
deserve, a normal relationship with food. As we talked through
these false beliefs, she came to the realization that, in spite of
understanding the concept of recovery, she didn't believe *she*
could obtain or maintain it. We started to put very specific, small,
and measurable goals in place. As each week went by and she met
her goals, she began seeing positive outcomes and believing she
could sustain them. With each small win, her motivation and trust
in the process continued to grow, eventually leading her to trust in
herself. Instead of beating herself up over the time it took to heal
her relationship to food, she shifted her perspective to see that her
ability to remain committed to recovery exemplified her resilience.
There was absolutely nothing wrong with her. Sara is now living a
life free of the daily battles with her food and continues to use the
tools she learned to improve her relationship with her body.

*"Nobody stays recovered unless the life they have created is
more rewarding and satisfying than the one they left behind."*
—Anne Fletcher, Sober for Good: New Solutions for Drinking
Problems—Advice from Those Who Have Succeeded

Make Time for Your Values

In chapter 2, you identified your values as a critical component of the ACT approach. Your current relationship to food has most likely consumed a great deal of your energy, focus, and time. As such, it has infringed upon the things that are truly important and bring you joy.

When Sara contacted me, she spoke about wanting to find something to keep her motivated in her recovery. Part of her weekly goal was to integrate back in the activities that were important to her well-being, but had fallen by the wayside due to work and general exhaustion. Eventually, she started stepping out of her comfort zone and began trying new things such as playing tennis and painting. She was surprised by how much she enjoyed these new hobbies, which improved her energy and decreased her general feelings of exhaustion.

Knowing what your values are provides you with an alternative path to bingeing. Taking ownership of this is key. It is up to you and you alone to make time to uphold your values. If you do, you are much more likely to maintain your recovery and, eventually, eradicate your binge eating. At the moment, it may feel difficult to identify more than just a few or any values at all. Most likely, the reason for this is that your struggle with disordered eating has preoccupied so much of your headspace that it is clouding over or completely blocking out the good things in your life. What do you think the value you have placed on your food and the thin ideal has brought to your life? What has it taken from you, and what have the costs of upholding this value been?

LIVING A VALUE-ORIENTED LIFE

The fact that you are holding this book is proof that you have hope that your life can be different. This means that some or many of the beliefs you currently have are not yielding the outcomes, or life, you desire. My assumption is that many of those detrimental beliefs are related to your self-worth and body image.

As discussed in chapter 1, our society places being thin high on the list of what constitutes success and/or desirability. It is part of our accepted social norms to glamorize thinness and ridicule fat. Sharing the details of our diet or attending exercise classes is also part of the way we relate to and connect with others.

Amid all of this, a person in recovery must begin to decide for themselves what will truly enrich their life. Is being thin an important value to you? If it feels inconceivable to let go of this desire, truly consider whether being thin really equates to happiness or success. Take a moment to think of a thin celebrity. When you have one in mind, think of what you know of their life. Has it been perfect? Has their low weight served to absolve them of unhappiness or struggle in one or more areas of their life?

I understand that even with this knowledge, a strong part of you may still be holding out hope that life will be better at a certain weight. I often have this debate with clients at the start of our work together, and, admittedly, I rarely win. The final response is usually, "Well, once I get there (the number on the scale they desire), I will stop dieting/focusing on my weight." I make it clear that I am not a clinician who can help them with weight loss; my work is around getting them to end their bingeing and improve their quality of life. As a result of their recovery, they may lose weight, but this can never be guaranteed. Understandably, they feel some disappointment and anxiety, fearing that they will never feel good in their body. To that end, I ask, "If you have not yet found success via diets, why not give this approach a chance?"

For the clients who have experienced being at a variety of sizes, including their goal weight, this concept is a bit easier to accept. I ask them to reflect on how happy they actually were at their ideal weight. Additionally, what was their day-to-day life like, what was different then versus now, and what did they have to do to get to that weight? Often, their responses are not as awe-inspiring as the initial vision of themselves at the lower weight. They'll remember how they had to miss out on plans with friends in order to spend hours at the gym. Or how on edge they were with their family because they had to prepare their own separate meal in order to follow their diet guidelines. Yes, they could fit into smaller clothing, but they still did not feel 100 percent comfortable in their bodies. And the ever-present fear of the weight returning became a self-fulfilling prophecy, as they eventually returned to or surpassed their previous weight.

In order to hit restart, I invite my clients to imagine a new vision for their life wherein they are living free of self-judgment and constant focus on their weight and food. In order to make this new vision a reality, they must let go of the old version of reality. Until they can let this version go, they will continue to compare and measure themselves against it. So much of our precious time is wasted striving for things that are meant to impress others or prove our value. Recovery is your way out of this limited perspective. As Carolyn Costin and Gwen Grabb state in their book, *8 Keys to Recovery from an Eating Disorder*, "When recovered, you no longer compromise health or betray your soul to look a certain way." What is waiting for you on the other side of recovery is a life lived aligned with your values, and the ability to make choices in honor of your soul.

THE POWER OF FEAR

Even though you may feel that you are 110 percent ready to end your binge eating, some part of you is not actually onboard. The brain has a mind of its own and usually works in ways that are favorable to your survival. Fear is an emotional mechanism to protect you from danger, but it can also cause a great amount of unnecessary suffering. Even in circumstances that are clearly beneficial, like getting promoted or winning the lottery, your mind can tarnish the experience by taking you through countless fear-based scenarios.

For example, if you got promoted, would your colleagues treat you differently because of your new role? Would they feel jealous of the pay raise, ultimately causing a divide that ends the friendship? And your boss's expectations of you would probably double, so how would you be able to meet them? Or, if you won the lottery, are you sure you would make the right decisions as to how to save/spend the money? Would you and your partner disagree on what to do with the money or if you should continue working? And how would it impact your friendships, children, extended family, etc.? Even though these questions bear some logic, the level of anxiety that is induced by the fear alters your ability to not only enjoy your good fortune, but also make decisions in a confident and decisive manner. Fear has the power to turn every option, decision, and route into the wrong one.

This is not to say that you must banish fear in order to become happy. Some amount of fear is part of a healthy decision-making process. But when its power over you becomes too strong, it can hold you back. If an outcome is uncertain or not guaranteed, fear will take the opportunity to fabricate a frightening scenario that gets at the heart of a person's conscious or subconscious fears. For someone in recovery, the unknown around what day-to-day life will actually look like can lead to a great amount of anxiety or foreboding scenarios. This is especially true for those who have struggled with disordered eating for as long as they can remember. They have no memory of what it felt like to trust their food choices or feel comfortable in their own body. Additionally, a realistic picture of what a healthy relationship with food might look like may be difficult to construct if they are surrounded by others who also have disordered relationships with food.

When we are uncertain of the outcome, we hold on, dig our heels in, and remain stuck in the same cycle. No matter how painful it may be, at least it is known and familiar. I explain to my clients that in order to heal their disordered eating, they will need to throw out their current life playbook and create a new one. Just like in football, depending on the opposing team (in this case, the trigger), some strategies or plays may not always work. But with each attempt, you can get closer to the goal.

New methods require a lot of patience, practice, and time to learn and execute, but once they're mastered, you will feel more in sync with your body and confident in your decisions. The part of you that likes consistency is going to push back hard, in any way it can. Hello, self-sabotage! One way around this is to get very clear on the reasons why you want recovery and how it correlates to your life's values.

ADDRESS YOUR TRIGGERS

Prior to beginning therapy, my clients complete an intake questionnaire about their life and their history with disordered eating. Their answers provide me with a sense of each person's overt and covert triggers for BED. Many express dissatisfaction in one or more areas of their life, in addition to their struggle with disordered eating. Particularly, they share feelings of unfulfillment in their relationships or careers. As we talk through these feelings, they often recognize they are not showing up authentically—not expressing their needs or doing what they are truly interested in or passionate about. Taking steps to address these important feelings is tremendously supportive to the process of ending bingeing and living the life you are meant to. In my first session with Mike, we addressed the purpose of his eating disorder and the intensity of feelings that lie beneath it:

I really do think it (the eating disorder) serves as an anesthetic to my depression and self-hatred. I feel like my life is run by fear— fear of the future, fear of time wasted and of life passing me by. I have countless regrets and am filled with shame. I know that if I am unable to address or come to terms with these feelings, I'm not sure I will be able to recover.

Mike's struggles with binge eating were clearly not only a result of external triggers. He was struggling with significant internal battles, including a lack of self-esteem, depression, and an unclear path or meaning in his life. He knew that it would be nearly impossible to recover if he did not heal the pain from the emotional wounds that the eating disorder helped to mollify. In order to create some separation from the intense judgments he had of himself, I encouraged him to name the different voices or parts of himself that represented those judgments and negative feelings. This helped him realize that one part of himself was speaking out of fear, not fact. Being able to categorize his thoughts also enabled him to remain more grounded when they popped up, accepting that they may never fully go away. The sting of negative internal commentary decreases when you can name the source, categorize it as inconsequential, and move on.

Here are a few names you can use to label the parts of yourself, or voices, that contribute to your internal dialogue:

- **Judgmental and/or unsupportive parts or voices:** the critic, eating disorder, the judge, the bully

- **Supportive parts or voices:** big sister/brother, the cheerleader, the empath, the nurturer, the reliable, authoritative parent

As you get better at recognizing which voice or part is saying what, you can do a better job of compartmentalizing or neutralizing them so they don't have the power to dictate emotions. To be clear, that voice is not you. It might sound like you and may have been around for as long as you can remember, but it is not you. In his book, *The Power of Now: A Guide to Spiritual Enlightenment*, spiritual teacher Eckhart Tolle refers to the identification with the unhappy, fearful self as the "fiction of the mind." There is a reason it exists and thinks the way it does, and it will never entirely go away. Sigmund Freud labeled these different parts as the id (instinctual thinker/rule breaker), superego (critic/rule follower), and ego (mediator/compromiser) and explained that we need all three working in tandem to flourish. When one becomes too powerful, your life will get out of balance.

In the treatment manual, *Erasing ED*, Sheira Kahn, MFT, and Nicole Laby, MFT, describe the relationship of these parts to eating disorders: "In all three eating disorder types, the body is the battleground in the conflict between the id and the superego, and food (restriction or consumption) is the ammunition. Each type of eating disorder is an expression of what is happening in the person's psyche. This is why it is important to conceptualize and treat eating disorders as mental illnesses with physical consequences, not as a physical illness with mental consequences."

Understanding your internal critic's purpose and motivation will help you put the commentary in perspective. By creating this cushion, you allow yourself to hear what the other parts of you have to say. For those whose critic has commanded center stage, it may take some time for the other parts of you to step in and grab the microphone.

ACCEPT THE PRESENT MOMENT

Why is it so hard to fully embrace recovery and make the choices you know are more in line with your values? When we resist our feelings in the present moment out of fear, we turn to anything that will numb or distract us from them. Even when you take steps to make intuitive decisions, eat your food mindfully, and sit with uncomfortable feelings, your habitual eating disorder behaviors may be waiting in the wings, eager for their chance to return and wreak havoc.

The critical voice pops up and tries to shut your recovery efforts down. It will use any tactic it can to talk you out of it, question your ability, and laugh at the audacity of you actually making a change. Regardless of the numerous circumstances you are able to change externally in your life (new job, city, relationship), this negative voice or part of you will follow. Again, naming this voice "the critic" is crucial to decreasing its power and providing you with the clarity of mind to make another choice. Within this dialogue is the pivotal moment when the decision is made to binge or not to binge. Thus, it is imperative that you create the internal space needed to begin decreasing the power of negative voices so they can become more manageable. By doing so, you can take advantage of the now freed-up space previously used by the critic to become more mindful of what your body needs in the moment.

Another way to practice distinguishing the parts is to journal the dialogues that take place in your mind. Through journaling, you can capture the critic's thoughts on paper and create a new dialogue for the other parts to speak. When all the different facets of you work together as a team, they are more capable of fostering the fulfilling life you desire—one that is built on a foundation of self-respect and unbreakable trust.

TAKE AN ACTIVE ROLE IN YOUR LIFE

During a recent session with John, he expressed his frustration around a recent increase in binge behaviors in spite of having several months of little to no bingeing. He pointed out how, on his recent solo trip to Costa Rica, he didn't binge at all and experienced hardly any urges to. I asked him to recall a time when he did have an urge and how he was able to avoid it. He reflected on a night where he got back to his hotel, pretty worn out from the day and feeling lonely. He ordered room service, and, after finishing his dinner, he contemplated ordering more. He decided against it and watched TV instead until he fell asleep.

I inquired further, "What was the dialogue in your mind at that moment when you decided against the binge?" He paused, and responded that another part of him chimed in, reminding him that he had a full day of activities tomorrow and wanted to feel his best to enjoy them and not miss out. His reliable, authoritative parent voice was strong in that moment, reminding him of the fun that was just around the corner, and that bingeing would be a hindrance. It was enough in that moment to convince him, and the urge to binge faded away.

John wondered how he could continue to disregard the urges to binge with such ease when not on vacation. We discussed how, in spite of how stressful work can be, he enjoys and looks forward to going in each day. So where was the catch? I pointed out how the feelings of loneliness were a trigger, and that the level of excitement and fun that awaited him the next day was enough to quell the urge to binge. We explored ways in which he could incorporate more joy into his life. He wrote out a list of more than 20 activities he enjoys doing, noting that they have always taken a back seat to work or other "more important" responsibilities. He recognized that if he truly wanted long-term recovery, he needed to incorporate these pleasures into his life and decrease his time at work.

John's story is not that unique. Many of my clients also struggle with boundaries around work or family responsibilities (or both), and can't seem to carve out a miniscule amount of time for themselves to relax or do something that brings them joy. Others may fear engaging in life, thinking that if they don't put themselves out there, they're saving themselves from pain, judgment, and disappointment. Additionally, they may feel worse if they try something new and then make a mistake, reinforcing their fear of being seen as a failure. Looking back, they reflect on the number of missed opportunities in their lives—things they were interested in but never pursued, all in the name of fear. They may feel this way because they've been negatively influenced by parents, teachers, or peers who did little to help build their self-esteem. Or they may have made these choices in order to keep others happy, stay in line with what was expected of them, or not "rock the boat." Many times, these clients will remark, "I have no idea what brings me joy; I've never considered it."

The practice of writing out what you value may be difficult on several levels. Some feel anxious naming what is important to them, for fear that something bad might happen as a result of claiming the significance. Others may feel safer being unhappy, always expecting the worst outcome. They tell themselves, "If I don't get my hopes up that something good will happen, I won't get too disappointed, and if something good does happen, I can be pleasantly surprised." That may be true, but then what does life look like between these events or circumstances? Constantly waiting for the bad and fearing the worst . . . is it even possible to truly enjoy the good when you quickly jump to worrying about when it will end?

Time to put pen to paper. You can either write out what your values are and how much of your current time is contributed to each value, or you can draw a pie chart to show how much time you devote to each value. Some values you might want to include are: family, friendships, intimate relationships, leisure/travel, volunteerism, spirituality, education, career/work, and health.

SMART Goals

Small, everyday decisions can help you attain goals that are in line with your values. Many of my clients struggle with intense perfectionism, believing that if they push themselves hard enough, they will eventually reach their goals, and subscribing to the old saying, "No pain, no gain." In our sessions, we typically refer to their critical voice as the drill sergeant or enforcer, using scare tactics as

THE IMPACT OF YOUR VALUES

In a pivotal session with my patient Riley, she realized the validity of her values and the significance of honoring them. She was thrilled to report that she had given two weeks' notice and bought a one-way airline ticket to Europe with plans to live abroad for one year. Riley was extremely frustrated with the reactions she was getting from family and friends about her decision. They could not understand why she would give up her high-paying job and great apartment to move abroad, with no real plan in place. Through tears, she explained that she had wanted to travel after high school, but feared how it would look to others. Instead, she went to college, attending an expensive school that made her parents intensely proud. Those four years ended up being the most difficult of her life. Her eating disorder grew out of control, and her depression nearly caused her to leave school. Eight years later, she still struggles with guilt, regret, and resentment toward herself and her family. She felt that her family's expectations—and her fear of being a disappointment—kept her from traveling abroad after high school. In hindsight, she can see how her eating disorder and depression worsened by going against her intuition and not making decisions in line with her values.

How might your values differ from your family's? Are you holding on to ones that are not your own? Riley knew what she wanted, yet was afraid to follow through. Upon reflection, she acknowledged that part of her did want to attend college. She feared feeling lonely, getting left behind, or missing out on experiences with her friends and peers. She felt stuck either way, but if she traveled and it had been a terrible experience, she would only have herself to blame. By choosing the "safer route," the blame could be shared. Ultimately, her desire to travel did not go away. Luckily, this time she is putting her values before fear and other people's expectations.

motivation. I will always suggest an alternative route. In her book *The Gifts of Imperfection*, Brené Brown, PhD, states, "Understanding the difference between healthy striving and perfectionism is critical to laying down the shield and picking up your life. Research shows that perfectionism hampers success. In fact, it's often the path to depression, anxiety, addiction, and life paralysis."

Based in CBT, the SMART system fosters a better rate of success in completing tasks that are in line with your goals. SMART stands for: Specific, Measurable, Achievable, Relevant, and Time-Limited. It encourages you to keep things simple by getting specific about a goal, then breaking it down in a way that can be tracked in order to foster motivation and celebrate success. Here is an example:

SMART GOAL: Reducing binge eating

- Specific: I want to bring my lunch to work every day this week.

- Measurable: Each time I do this, I will draw a star next to the day in my calendar.

- Achievable: I have enough groceries at home, and there is enough space in the fridge at work to make this possible.

- Relevant: By bringing my lunch, I will be less tempted to skip lunch or get triggered to binge on whatever food is around the office.

- Time-Limited: I plan to try this for one workweek (five days) and then reevaluate.

After you've written out your own SMART goals, write about why you chose the specific goals. Is your desire to meet them internally or externally driven? Are you hoping someone close to you will notice or acknowledge your progress? If these are goals you've had in the past, what has gotten in the way of accomplishing them?

Lastly, having a calendar that is easily accessible will help you stay on top of your goals by providing a realistic picture of your daily/weekly/monthly commitments. If you do not have one already, purchase a planner that is convenient to carry with you, or use an online scheduler that you can access via your cell phone and computer.

EXERCISE Goal Setting Activity—Miracle Day

The question below is a popular tool used in solution-focused therapy to help clients become clear on "the why" or reason for their goals, and to create a picture of what life would be like if they were able to reach their goals.

Question:

Imagine, when you go to sleep, a miracle happens and your problem has disappeared. When you wake up the next morning, you don't know the miracle happened, as you were fast asleep. What will be the first sign that tells you that the miracle has happened?

Response:

In your journal, write down how you see yourself moving through your day, having recovered from binge eating. Provide as much detail as possible. For example, if your initial response to the question was, "I would feel happy or content," what would that *exactly* look like? What would change internally and externally? What would remain the same? How would you talk to or engage with yourself? What emotions would be present? Consider how you could start to integrate some of the changes you'd make after the miracle, now. What feelings arise as you consider this?

Getting Unstuck

Even though you've done the work to identify what you value and what your goals are, you may be feeling stuck in other ways, or overwhelmed by the possibility of changing your behavior.

Since our brains are still wired to help us survive caveman-like conditions, they have functions that no longer serve us. For instance, our brains hold on to negative information in order to protect us from future danger. Rick Hanson describes this archaic trait in his book, *The Buddha's Brain*, providing reasons why our minds hold on to positive moments like Teflon and negative moments like Velcro. Luckily, there are ways we can retrain the brain. Here are some strategies for getting out of your head:

- Increase happiness: In order to train your brain to register and recall positive memories, you must actively seek out ways to increase your ability to feel happy.

- Choose love over hate: It's very simple to ask yourself if what you are saying or doing is being done out of love or spite. By using self-compassion and radical acceptance, you can more easily move out of hate and into love.

- Increase mindfulness: When you pause and become present in the moment, you put yourself in charge of your decision-making, instead of relying on automatic thoughts, behaviors, or reflexes.

PRACTICE POSITIVE ALTERNATIVES

When implementing new coping mechanisms, you must have a realistic expectation that they will not cancel out the urge to binge right away. By trying out a variety of coping tools, you can sharpen your self-care tools and increase your ability to handle triggers, eventually replacing food as your only or most soothing option. When we get into the habit of taking care of ourselves in a multitude of ways, food naturally become less and less of a go-to over time. Committing to practicing new methods of self-care, and letting go of the guilt of emotional eating will set you up for success. Further, focusing on adding new coping mechanisms, rather than subtracting others, is more realistic, and less likely to lead to rebellion in the long run.

CHECK IN WITH YOUR SPIRITUAL SIDE

Your experience with or perspective of spirituality has likely been impacted by factors such as your religion, where you grew up, and your family and/or peers. Regardless of whether you follow a certain religion, spirituality can be a strong contributing factor to fostering mental and emotional equanimity. If you've struggled with religion, have turned away from it entirely, or have never believed in one, cultivating a relationship with faith, spirituality, or rituals will be propitious to your recovery.

> *"The secret of change is to focus all of your energy not on fighting the old, but on building the new."*
> — *Dan Millman*, Way of the Peaceful Warrior

The Oxford Living Dictionaries defines spirituality as "the quality of being concerned with the human spirit or soul as opposed to material or physical things." This definition applies greatly to your process of shifting focus from the external to your intuition—your authentic feelings and needs. One way to create a ritual around this would be to clean out your closet for "spring cleaning" or at the start of each new season, and donate things you no longer need to a local shelter. Another way to deepen your spirituality could be to prioritize being in nature. Spending time outdoors has been shown to decrease stress cortisol levels, depression, and anxiety while increasing feelings of awe, concentration, creative thinking, and overall connection to one's surroundings.

A great way to bridge your mindfulness practice with the calming benefits of nature is to do a walking meditation. There is no right or wrong way to do this; it can even be done during your walk to work. The important thing is that you use the time to become mindful and present in your current experience.

As you walk, begin to focus on your steps. Slow your pace and become more aware of and intentional with your steps. Notice your breath and how the air feels in your lungs and on your skin. Focus on how you place your foot on the ground and how you lift your foot off the ground, switching from left to right. Notice your breath, and allow any thoughts that arise to just pass on by, as you continue to slowly take mindful steps.

Elevate Your Mood

Carving out time to engage in things that will keep you in an affirmative mood will facilitate the more challenging facets of healing your BED. This can be a delicate balance to reach, but it's crucial to maintaining motivation. In addition to the tools and techniques that address how you can mentally reduce stress and urges to binge, recovery must also involve integrating more positive activities in your life. You may be less inclined to do these things as you focus your time on what you assume to be the more productive pieces of your recovery. Yet, this component of self-care is just as important. Your mind-set will eventually come around to this as you begin to experience the shifts and overall benefits to your life.

WHAT DO YOU ENJOY?

Due to the eating disorder's all-encompassing nature, you may be doing very few things that bring you joy. Mindfulness can also be a tool to help you reconnect with your creativity. For many of us, the notion of "I'm not artistic" has kept us from engaging in activities that provide relaxation and a different way to connect with ourselves. For others, creativity may be blocked due to the perfectionistic voice relegating it to conditions that must be just right, or a voice that says you can only engage in fun activities after you finish the 100+ tasks on your to-do list!

MOVEMENT AND EXERCISE

Most likely, you already know that there are many health benefits to exercise. In addition to decreasing stress and susceptibility to illness and disease, it improves mental clarity, increases energy, and supports better sleep quality. Depending on your history with exercise, this may be a very sensitive issue that should be put on hold for now. But if you have ever had a positive experience with exercise, consider incorporating it into your life, solely as a way to boost your mood. From this mind-set, consider if that will mean increasing your level of movement (walking/stretching) or attending a class, such as yoga or dance. Again, the only intention behind this must be the positive mental health benefit (for now). We will get more in-depth on the subject of exercise in chapter 6.

SLEEP AND REST

Just as important to your health and well-being, if not more so, is the quantity and quality of your sleep. Rest plays a huge role in your life and recovery, namely your mood and hunger levels. Similar to your relationship with food, the importance you give sleep may have been impacted by those around you. Culturally, our attitude is something along the lines of, "You can sleep when you're dead," which clearly promotes an unhealthy value of balance. Just as we manipulate our bodies to eat a certain way, we push them to exhaustion time and again. In an effort to improve the information we are given regarding fostering not only physical health, but mental health as well, doctors Dan Siegel and David Rock created a tool called *The Healthy Mind Platter*. This tool details seven activities we should be engaging our mind in on a daily basis to improve brain matter and increase overall well-being. Of the seven (sleep time, physical time, focus time, time in, down time, play time, and connecting time), three are focused around slowing down and allowing for rest in order to recharge and boost our brain power. Consider how you can prioritize sleep and rest, especially as you work on your recovery.

EXERCISE   Creating a Self-Care Plan

"When you discover something that nourishes your soul and brings joy, care enough to make room for it in your life."
—Jean Shinoda Bolen, MD

Create a list of at least 20 self-care-oriented activities. Starting tomorrow, use the SMART goal system (page 59) to integrate at least one self-care activity into your daily schedule. For example, begin your day with a mindful moment before you step out of bed. Decide how much time you will dedicate to it and how you will track it.

Journal about your experiences, and have questions prepared that you can easily complete. For example: Did I have any setbacks? What can I do differently tomorrow? Have I experienced any benefits from the goals I've set thus far?

Continued Practice

In this chapter, we delved into how important it is to make sure your goals are aligned with your values in order to have success in obtaining them and eventually changing your life. We discussed the powerful roles of our myriad parts and what happens when they fall out of balance. The emotion of fear and our desire to remain safe, regardless of whether the resulting behavior is actually good for us, tends to be a significant motivating factor behind the pessimistic dialogues in our mind.

In the following chapters, you will

- learn how your relationship with your body impacts your ability to intuitively eat.

- discover what part your emotions play in your hunger and decisions around food.

- find out how you can implement the tools and strategies for healing and make them work for you.

CHAPTER FOUR

Listening to Your Body

Most likely, your disordered eating began in part because of negative thoughts or beliefs about your body. The thoughts were progressively reinforced and became ingrained as you engaged in repeated efforts to control or alter your body by dieting. Now, these thoughts are triggers for binge eating. In order to free yourself from BED, you must make significant changes in how you relate to and care for your body. The relationship you have with your body is even more important than the one you have with your food. Listening to your body may seem like a foreign concept or, conversely, something you feel you are already doing excessively. I received the following email from Jenny, 25, who was tired of living her life hating her body:

> *I don't quite know where to begin here, but I am coming to you for help to regain control of my relationship with food. I have struggled with binge eating and body image issues my whole life, but I feel like right now I'm in the middle of a very bad "episode" and can't seem to get myself out of*

it like I normally do. This issue affects my daily life and productivity at work, and I am willing to do whatever is necessary to get control of this. I have never really had a positive relationship with my body, and I feel like my insecurities over the past few years have increased. Getting dressed in the morning is like a merciless battle I must suffer through every day, usually requiring at least an hour to try on multiple things in order to feel remotely comfortable before I walk out the door. I want to be able to speak more positively to myself, love myself and my body. I just have no idea how to make that happen. I am tired of feeling so self-conscious and judgmental of myself and others. I feel terrible about the critiques I make of other people's bodies, yet cannot stop comparing my body to everyone else's every time I enter a room. I know that all of this negativity and insecurity impacts my social life and relationships, particularly with my parents and boyfriend. It is difficult to imagine actually feeling good in my body, but I know something must change. I don't want to live my life hating my body anymore.

When we met, Jenny told me that she discovered intuitive eating while doing an online search and had had success in decreasing her binge eating using its principles. In spite of her progress, she felt frustrated that the bingeing hadn't stopped completely and the discomfort in her body remained just as strong. Her goals included (1) working on improving her body image, (2) learning how not to take her frustration out on the people she loves when she is struggling, and (3) decreasing the impact body image has on her thoughts, actions, and ability to enjoy life.

I expressed to Jenny how encouraging it was that she acknowledged the significance of her goals and had already begun to practice intuitive eating. Her intention to work specifically on improving her body image will serve her in many ways. It will not only help to heal her disordered eating, but it will also bring a great deal of contentment and ease to her life. In some ways, improving body image can feel entirely separate from ending binge eating. Thus, this part of recovery often progresses slower and, in some ways, is never entirely complete, as your body continuously evolves during your lifetime. Being patient with yourself and having reasonable expectations about your body image will help you to stay on track.

As you go through this chapter, you will learn more about cultivating body acceptance, as well as the science behind why the desire to control your weight is the fuel for binge eating.

EXERCISE Basic Body Scan

Many people struggling with disordered eating associate their bodies with feelings of perpetual disappointment, admonishment, and condemnation. In order to change this association, you must begin to connect with your body in new and different ways. This will require you to slow down in order to focus on listening to and addressing what your body needs. As you do so, you will start to notice how much your body and mind are connected and impact one another. When one becomes out of balance, eventually so will the other. For a person struggling with an eating disorder, the body is the innocent victim of the critic's wrath. The critic is focused on perfection versus self-acceptance, continually trying to manipulate and control the body in order to achieve an "acceptable" shape or weight.

Taking mindful breaks will help you foster a healthy connection with your body. Use the following breathing exercise to zero in on your current physical state and release tension in your body:

Begin by sitting in a comfortable upright position. Take one to two deep breaths, and just allow yourself to be present in your body. Starting at the top of your head, notice any feelings of tightness or tension. Make your way down to your jaw, neck, and shoulders. If you feel any tightness, allow yourself to stretch; roll your shoulders back and relax your jaw. Take deep breaths, and as you do, direct each breath to an area of tension. Continue to make your way down your body to your back, lower back, hips, and buttocks. Move down your arms, wrists, and fingers. Again, check in with your breath and stretch or adjust any part of the body that feels tight. As you go down your legs, through the knees, shins, and down to your feet, feel as if you are allowing any remaining bits of tension to flow out through your toes. Take another one to two deep breaths, and take note of how you feel now versus when you started.

"Our minds are like politicians; they make stuff up, they twist the truth. Our minds are masters at blame, but our bodies . . . our bodies don't lie."
—Geneen Roth, Women Food and God: An Unexpected Path to Almost Everything

You, In Your Body

Is it actually possible to accept or even like our bodies if they do not fit our current idealized image of beauty? In order to reach your goal of ending binge eating and living a better life, you must address your body image. When your mind is clouded by critiques, self-recriminations, and guilt, you are disconnected from your body and likely feel hopeless that your relationship to your body will ever change. By decreasing the judgmental chatter in your mind, you will be able to tap into what your body actually needs with regard to food and exercise. For this to really work, you must go all in and put an end to the restrictive, punitive mind-set. Holding out to see if this approach actually works with the plan that you can just go on another diet will impair you in the moments where you must challenge yourself. Relying on the possibility of returning to or trying a new diet is like the "Get Out of Jail Free" card in Monopoly, which will take you back to "GO," restarting the cycle again and again. Instead, take a leap of faith and use whatever has resonated with you thus far to jump in with *both* feet, not just one!

Why can the idea of starting another diet be so enticing? We are taught (directly or indirectly) to conform our bodies to society's standards of beauty. As infants and young children, we did not register a certain weight as beautiful or ugly. As we grew, our exposure to the media and the adults around us began to inform our understanding of our bodies and what is perceived as good or acceptable. This distinction of good versus bad often becomes fodder for bullying or teasing by siblings and peers. Unfortunately, just as common as stories of peer-to-peer bullying are memories of seemingly unintentional comments or actions made by parents, family, teachers, and doctors.

When I asked Jenny if she had any memories relating to her body, she swiftly recalled a comment her father made when she was 14, while at their family's summer cottage. As she was about to head out to meet her cousins for an afternoon of swimming at the nearby lake, her father said, "Looks like it's time to get a bigger swimsuit." She froze in that moment, flooded with embarrassment and body shame. From then on, she felt uncomfortable being around others at the lake and began wearing a T-shirt over her swimsuit. The following summer, she began making excuses to avoid going swimming. The year after, she decided to get a summer job so she could skip out on the summer getaways altogether. Her family felt hurt by her withdrawal and regularly pressured her to join them. Like clockwork, tension would grow between Jenny and her parents in the few weeks leading up to summer vacation. She could not summon the courage to tell her family the real reason why she was upset, forcing herself to keep her now full-fledged eating disorder a secret. Even in our therapy session, she acknowledged how uncomfortable it was for her to share this memory with me, as she did not want to blame her father for her eating disorder and wished it was something she could have just "gotten over."

THE TRIALS OF ADOLESCENCE

It's rare that someone can pinpoint the moment when they began to lose trust in their body. In addition to being inundated by society's ideals regarding food and weight, many people can recall several damaging experiences that impacted the development of their negative body image. Some of the most common situations that may have led to negative body image include traumatic events, participating in highly competitive sports, being transgender, or growing up with parents or other role models who modeled body-mistrust or body-hatred behavior. The experience of our bodies developing through adolescence is rife with unpleasantness, to put it lightly. On top of the expectations around academics or extracurricular activities, we are also pressured to begin dating and decide on our future paths. We go through significant hormonal changes that impact our mental and physical states, yet education around this is usually minimal. And frequently, instead of helping, the adults around us only add to this awkward and confusing time. Depending on your parents' relationship with their bodies, their reactions to your development may have been largely influenced by their own negative experiences during their childhood or teenage years. If they were bullied for their weight, they may overcompensate in a variety of ways in an effort to shield their children from experiencing the same pain.

The way a mother introduces the concept of menstruation to her daughter (if there is an introduction at all) can be indicative of the relationship she has with her own body. Were these pubescent changes talked about in your family? If they were, was it from a negative or supportive viewpoint?

Additionally, adolescence is a time when we attempt to create our identities—to see where we fit among our peers while still retaining our uniqueness and independence. As the brain is still developing at this time, teens are operating out of the amygdala, the region of the brain that is responsible for emotions. This part of the brain is responsible for impulsive reactions, like fear and anger, and gives little importance to long-term consequences. Many of our current beliefs about ourselves originated during this time, when emotions were intense and the only possible responses were fight or flight. As a teen, did you speak up or act out, or were your thoughts and feelings kept private?

BODY ACCEPTANCE

It may feel very difficult to imagine accepting your body as it is right now. When I discuss this with clients, their responses are often filled with fear and anxiety around what could happen as a result of this drastic mind-set change. For so long, their belief has been, "I will be able to accept my body once I lose weight." They know they want to make a change, but they can't imagine how to be happy with their current body without a major epiphany or transformation.

You might have noticed that I have not directly addressed the issue of weight in the preceding chapters. This is not to suggest that weight isn't an important factor in healing binge eating. On the contrary, it is likely the most significant cause of your binge eating and current body image. Therefore, if you are truly ready to stop binge eating, you must start accepting or respecting your body, regardless of your current weight. I can almost hear the alarm bells going off, telling you that this approach isn't for you. I understand how disconcerting this can feel, but hopefully by now your interest has been piqued enough to give this a try and keep going. The most common fears I hear are "If I try to accept my body, my weight will spiral out of control and there will be no going back" and "Is this just me giving up on myself and my body?" I will address these fears later in this chapter, but know this: Ending the battle with your weight sets you free from the fear-based thoughts that keep you bingeing and letting the number on a scale dictate your life. In fact, dieting or following any restrictive mind-set in order to control your weight has kept you stuck in more ways than just the bingeing.

BODY IMAGE ADVOCACY

Recent movements toward body acceptance and body positivity have been born out of the frustration caused by unrealistic and detrimental ideals of beauty. In her book, *Eating in the Light of the Moon*, Anita Johnston writes, "Why has a naturally masculine shape (broad shoulders, no waist, narrow hips, flat belly) become the ideal for the female body? Why is it that those aspects of a woman's body that are most closely related to her innate female power, the capacity of her belly, hips, and thighs to carry and sustain life, are diminished in our society's version of a beautiful woman?"

But how does one go about accepting their body, especially after years or decades of doing the exact opposite? Similar to mindful eating, you will need to pause and be curious in order to hear your body's needs regarding rest, movement, and hunger. Additionally, you must pay attention to what you are thinking and saying about your body. Consider the observations you make when you stand in front of a mirror. What does the typical commentary consist of? How long have you been thinking and feeling these things about your body or certain parts of it? Now, consider saying some of those things to a friend or your child regarding their body. Did you have a mental/physical response to just my *suggestion* of that? Imagine the quality of relationship you would have if you said those things to them on a daily basis, for years. Begin to track your thoughts, and work on adding a compassionate response to your internal dialogue. Responses could include, "This thought or judgment is not helpful to me or my body," or "I may not like how my [body part] looks, but I do like my [body part]."

In addition to changing the way you talk to yourself about your body, here is a list of ideas to improve your body image:

- Get rid of your scale (more on this in chapter 6)
- Place notes of positive affirmations on mirrors, in your phone, or in your day planner
- Get rid of clothes that no longer fit
- Buy new clothes that you feel good in
- Do not engage in diet talk with others
- Get massages, visit a day spa or steam room
- Do yoga (at home or in a class setting)
- Take a bath
- Dance (at home, in a class)
- Lovingly apply lotion to your body after shower/bath
- Paint your nails or get a manicure/pedicure

IMPROVING SELF-ESTEEM AND IDENTITY

A client, Rachel, shared a recent talk she had with her close colleague and friend. He told her how concerned he was that she constantly expressed feeling stressed and overwhelmed. He noticed how she would continually put the needs of others before her own and would rarely ask for or accept help. In spite of being very well-liked by colleagues and her boss, Rachel never seemed to really accept their positive feedback and would push herself even harder. He worried how this was impacting her health (he was unaware of her binge eating) and encouraged her to work on her self-esteem in order to improve her well-being.

In our session, Rachel expressed that she felt embarrassed by her colleague's observations, particularly the comment he made about her low self-esteem. She knew that what he said was true, but it was a surprise to her that it was apparent to those around her. We explored where this need to exceed expectations and handle everything on her own came from. Rachel acknowledged that it had been present in each job she'd had, and had been noted by previous bosses as well.

We then talked about her academics: she got straight As in college and was active in many clubs. I questioned where this drive to excel came from. Was it an expectation held by her teachers or parents? Rachel did not feel much pressure from her parents, but thought it was an expectation she imposed upon herself. In considering further, she recalled that it started all the way back in grade school. She was in the 5th grade and was repeatedly being teased by a boy in her class about her weight. He was the only one who teased her or made any comments about her body, but she felt so self-conscious about it that she never told a teacher or her parents about the bullying, so it went on for years. Rachel believed she had to find other ways to stand out and distract attention from her body size. In conjunction with the development of her eating disorder (which started out as anorexia, then morphed into bulimia), she threw herself into academics as a way to feel in control of her identity.

Many clients can relate to Rachel in their desire to claim a persona as an effort to distract or minimize the possible judgment by others around their weight. For those who do make their weight a form of their identity, weight gain due to injury, pregnancy, or yo-yo dieting can cause a tremendous amount of mental anguish. In either case, letting go of this facet of your identity can feel very daunting. Yet, gradually creating a new identity that is more in line with your current values will contribute to your overall self-worth and well-being.

HEALTH AT EVERY SIZE

One of the movements supporting body acceptance and autonomy is the Health at Every Size® (HAES) paradigm. Its premise is
based on creating a more respectful and compassionate approach
to a person's overall health. It honors the fact that our bodies are
unique and are not supposed to fit one type of mold. HAES advo-
cates believe in moving the focus off of thinness as a necessary
component of health, and instead encourage healthy behaviors
irrespective of weight.

In a keynote address at a conference on body diversity, activist,
author, and HAES advocate Virgie Tovar stated: "When people say
they want to lose weight, they often mean, 'I want to be respected.
I want to be loved. I want to be seen. I want liberation from fear
and self-loathing.' Weight loss culture will never give us those
things because it is founded on fear/hate-based systems like sex-
ism, racism, classism and ableism . . . And at the end of the day, we
still feel empty, because worthiness ain't out there; it is something
that rises from within. Worthiness is something we cultivate from
a deep place at the center of our being."

If you study the history of our society's preoccupation with
women's bodies, you'll see that society has predominantly preferred a curvy figure. In the book *Beyond a Shadow of a Diet*,
Judith Matz and Ellen Frankel address how this body ideal
changed in 1965 when the fashion magazine *Vogue* popularized
the ultra-thin ideal by putting the model Twiggy on its cover. The
new ideal "encouraged women to take up less space in the world
rather than more, to be weak rather than powerful, and to be concerned about the minutiae of their bodies . . . . The new ideal body
encouraged competition between women and an obsession with
being thin as the mark of true success." This obsession has fueled
the diet industry, as the decision to diet is a result of feeling inad-
equate in our bodies. Healing and changing this mind-set will take
work, including educating yourself about modern body diversity

movements and looking at scientific research regarding health and weight with a discerning eye. But to heal your body image, the solution cannot be weight loss.

HAES and other body positive movements want to bring an end to the way so many men and women are putting their lives on hold until their weight is deemed acceptable. Often, size—not ability—keeps people from engaging in physical activity and other positive pursuits, as they worry that they might be judged, or believe the stigma that they are unable to do certain things.

EXERCISE   What Do You Like About Yourself?

Our tendency to focus on the negative keeps us from seeing situations fairly or objectively. In *The Happiness Advantage*, Shawn Anchor writes, "happiness is a choice, happiness is an advantage, happiness spreads." Regarding the debate between seeing the glass as half full or half empty, he believes that it doesn't really matter how you see it as long as you know there is a pitcher nearby. If your perspective on a situation is negatively skewed, that's fine, as long as you have some trust that your life will provide you with other ways to refill your glass.

For this exercise, reflect on what you currently like about your life. What characteristics do you like about yourself in particular? Write down your positive traits and strengths. If it is too difficult to think of things, ask someone you trust to tell you what they most appreciate about you. Write about how your positive traits and strengths can support you in living your life more in line with the values you identified in chapter 3 (page 48).

Understanding Your Body's Cues

In chapter 1, we briefly discussed what drives us to eat or overeat when we're hungry and when we're not. In order to make food decisions that are attuned to your body, you will need to recognize the cues your body provides you. By listening to these signals, you will make choices that will enable you to feel more satiated and satisfied in the long run.

ARE YOU HUNGRY?

For many people struggling with BED, hunger cues are thwarted by the restrict-binge-restrict cycle. Your hunger cues are your body's way of providing you the information you need to keep functioning in homeostasis, or in a stable range. Differentiating your cues will help you eat intuitively and make healthy decisions about what and how much to eat.

When a client has difficulty identifying their hunger cues, I walk them through the 10-point hunger scale—starting at zero, which indicates no hunger at all or a state of complete fullness, and going up to 10, which indicates extreme hunger or starvation. As you experience feeding yourself intuitively, you will get a better sense of how much you need to eat at various points of the hunger scale in order to feel satiated. Again, there is no perfection in this, but in time it will become second nature.

Intuitive eating also requires you to discover what types of food you actually do and do not like. For example, a particular client realized that she really did not like the taste of the energy bars she was eating on a daily basis. Half the time after eating a bar, a binge would follow. When she recognized that she was not satisfying her hunger cues, she decided to trade her bars for peanut butter and jelly sandwiches.

THE MYTH OF RESTRICTION

Understanding what goes on in your body when you lose weight will help shed light on what causes the yo-yo effect of the weight loss–weight gain cycle. When you lose weight as a result of cutting back on either your total calories or certain foods, your body will think it is being starved, which triggers the survival part of your brain. Historically, to survive famines, your body needed to be able to adjust its functioning in order to conserve energy. When you lose weight, you also lose muscle, and your metabolism will begin to decrease in order to conserve the stored energy. Additionally, your appetite will increase in hopes of rebuilding energy levels. When the weight is regained, instead of your metabolism returning to its initial speed, it will stay at that decreased level. The vast majority of people will regain the weight they lost and often gain more. The following statistics come from the Eating Disorder Hope website:

- At any given time, more than half of all teenage girls and one-third of all teenage boys are using restrictive measures to lose weight.
- Out of the 46 percent of 9- to 11-year-olds that diet occasionally or often, 82 percent of their families practice restriction-based diets.
- In a recent survey of females on one college campus, 91 percent reported that they had some history with dieting, and 22 percent said that they dieted often or constantly.
- 95 percent of all people who diet will regain the lost weight in one to five years.
- 35 percent of normal dieters progress to pathological dieting, and 20 to 25 percent of pathological dieters progress to eating disorders.
- On any given day, 25 percent of American men and 45 percent of American women are dieting.

The process of eating intuitively will involve putting your needs first. From planning and prepping food to speaking up to family and friends when deciding where to eat. We will go into more detail on how to make these changes in chapter 6.

ARE YOU FULL?

Typically, it's easier to recognize hunger cues than it is to recognize fullness cues. As you become more comfortable in honoring the hunger cues and mindfully eating, the fullness cues will become more distinctive. Further, as you begin to recognize where your hunger falls on the hunger scale, you will be able to recognize at what point you feel comfortably satiated. The actual feeling of fullness can hold different meanings for someone with an eating disorder, signaling that they have over-indulged or failed at their restrictive diet and triggering unpleasant emotional feelings. They may also feel bloated in spite of not eating a large amount and become angry with their body and the feelings of discomfort. Conversely, some may welcome the feeling of fullness as a soothing comfort. This may be the only time in their day that they feel satisfied instead of achingly empty or unfulfilled.

ACKNOWLEDGING CRAVINGS

Cravings are another type of signal your body will give you in order to help you feel satiated and content. By acknowledging your cravings, you will be in a better position to eat more mindfully and stop when full. In order to honor them as much as possible, you must have access to a variety of foods at home and at work. That way, you can avoid trying to soothe a craving with something other than what you actually want. By giving your body what will truly "hit the spot," you may avoid feeling hungry again

HUNGER SCALE	FEELING
1	Starving and feeling weak/dizzy
2	Very hungry, irritable, low energy, large amounts of stomach growling
3	Pretty hungry, stomach is beginning to growl
4	Beginning to feel hungry
5	Satisfied, neither hungry nor full
6	Slightly full/pleasantly full
7	Slightly uncomfortable
8	Feeling stuffed
9	Very uncomfortable, stomachaches
10	So full you feel sick

shortly after or triggering a binge. This means prioritizing regular trips to the grocery store and buying things that you know you like.

Understandably, this suggestion may bring up feelings of anxiety. I am essentially encouraging you to fill your cabinets and refrigerator with foods that have historically triggered you to binge. Again, breaking out of the cycle means doing things in a different way. It will not go perfectly at first, but allowing yourself to eat what you are craving in the moment is key to becoming an attuned eater.

For my client Ben, eating bread would usually lead to a binge, as bread had been a forbidden food in his household as a child. In order to release this negative association, I suggested he start stocking a loaf of bread in his freezer. We also talked through the different ways he could use the bread as part of a meal. In spite of wanting desperately to let this food fear go, he was extremely anxious, presuming that, frozen or not, he would finish the bread in one, two days max. In order to motivate him, we discussed one of his values, which was a desire to be in a serious relationship. One of his fears of being serious with someone would be that she would pick up on his rigidity around food, especially if she came to his house and saw how little food he had stocked in his fridge and cabinets. His desire for a serious relationship helped him to push past this fear, and, as a result, he now has no problem keeping fresh bread in his house.

AM I ADDICTED TO FOOD?

Many people wonder if they're addicted to food, expressing how much they have always loved food and the amount of time they spend thinking about it. There are various viewpoints on this issue. You are biologically engineered to want food and to enjoy consuming it. Unlike drugs and alcohol, you would not survive if you abstained from food completely. More so, your body does not respond well if you try to restrict it or non-intuitively manage it. Yet, when following a diet, the body may respond in an addict-like manner. It may crave certain foods, and the urge for them may become overwhelmingly intense. Similar to addictive substances, food distracts you from an emotional trigger, and, eventually, eating to cope becomes a habit that feels impossible to break.

EXERCISE Checking in with Your Body Before You Eat

After disregarding your hunger cues for a significant amount of time, you may have some difficulty hearing what it is that your body wants to eat. The following question from the book *Beyond a Shadow of a Diet*, by Judith Matz and Ellen Frankel, may be helpful in improving your ability to make intuitive food choices when you feel stuck or overwhelmed:

"If I had a magic wand to tell me what exactly would be the most appetizing and satiating meal, what would it be?"

This question can also help you distinguish what part of you is chiming in (eating disorder voice or recovery voice) and help you feel more confident that you are making decisions in line with your recovery. Ultimately, by checking in with your body more consistently, you will be prepared to go into the decision-making process with a mind-set that is more attuned to your needs.

The Necessity of Nutrition

The concept of clean eating or maintaining a vegetarian diet seems to present a way of eating that will simplify things and keep you in pristine health. I approach this with clients by first discrediting the idea that so many people are able to eat clean or healthy *all of the time*. Many of my clients who proclaim to be or are perceived as clean eaters by family and friends do not eat this way, yet they keep this a secret out of shame or in an effort to preserve their identity. No one eats "perfectly," because there is no perfect way of eating! Food was not meant to have a value or bearing on your self-worth or identity. It is meant to be enjoyed and to give your body fuel. When you don't eat what your body requires, you will experience gastrointestinal pain, allergies, acid reflux, etc. Recognizing what foods and what meal times work for you is a process that's continuously evolving. The desire to categorize foods as good versus bad or forbidden will only serve to keep food in power.

In order for my clients to overcome their anxiety around foods they've deemed forbidden, I encourage them to start keeping these foods in their house. Many balk at the idea, thinking that it will create more urges and opportunities to binge. It may in the beginning, but evicting those foods from the house won't stop the bingeing from occurring, either. To regain your power over food,

SUBSTANCE ABUSE

It is not uncommon for someone to struggle with drugs and alcohol in addition to binge eating. In a 2003 study titled *Food for Thought: Substance Abuse and Eating Disorders*, the National Center on Addiction and Substance Abuse at Columbia University reported that "up to 50% of individuals with eating disorders abused alcohol or illicit drugs, compared to 9% of the general population." Both substance abuse and eating disorders share similar risk factors, including depression, anxiety, low self-esteem, and vulnerability during times of transition or increased stress. Similar to the binge, the urge to use drugs is impulsive and compulsive, and is often done in secret in tandem with binge eating.

Like bingeing, drugs provide a physical high by increasing the release of dopamine and blocking its reuptake. There is an initial flood of feel-good feelings followed by a sense of calm and numbness. If the drug is taken consistently, the tolerance level increases, requiring greater quantities to obtain the same high. Similarly, as binges become more frequent, the "high" gradually lessens as the pain/cost of the behaviors increases. It is often at this point that someone reaches out for help.

Recovery becomes even more difficult if these behaviors go hand in hand. Alcohol and drugs, such as marijuana, serve as numbing agents to the critical/perfectionist internal voice and enable the urge to binge. Typically, clients who struggle with both binge eating and substance addiction will make progress in decreasing one, only to have the other increase in frequency. If this is something you are struggling with, it is important to take into consideration how each of these behaviors is triggered and what level of abstinence from drugs and alcohol is doable as you work on your BED recovery.

If you are considering getting support to address substance use, I recommend attending a 12-step meeting such as Alcoholics Anonymous (AA) or Narcotics Anonymous (NA). These drop-in meetings are free and provide you with peer support, a sense of community, and the option of a sponsor for one-on-one guidance and accountability. If you do not struggle with alcohol or drug abuse, but someone in your life did or does, I recommend attending an Adult Children of Alcoholics (ACA) or Co-dependents Anonymous (CoDA) meeting.

you must face the rules you set for yourself in an attempt to gain control. Surrendering to the assumption, "I cannot have it in sight or I will binge eat it," only fuels your fear. Each minute, hour, or day that you do not binge on the food will help you feel stronger and truly in control.

SPLURGING, MINDFULLY

A component of binge eating is a feeling of rebelliousness or an "I deserve it" attitude. Do you imagine this going away once you are eating intuitively? I can safely say that it will not. Even people who do not struggle with disordered eating will choose to over-eat or splurge on meals, snacks, or desserts from time to time. The difference is that, for them, it will not be followed by hours or days of regret or extreme physical discomfort and pain. Instead of thinking, "Screw it—my day is ruined," and eating more than feels comfortable, those who do not suffer from BED will feel satiated, and their thoughts will not linger on the food. Since they trust their body, they know that it will balance itself out.

EXERCISE   Creating a Realistic Mood Board

Do you struggle with constantly comparing yourself to others? When you walk into a café, do your thoughts automatically go to how your body measures up against the other people in the room? My clients express how they often feel like they are the heaviest people in the room and will feel a sense of relief when they are thinner than those around them. Additionally, they feel a compulsion or obsession to follow people on social media who demonstrate the ideal clean eating lifestyle and post images of their food and/or bodies.

Assess the magazines you subscribe to and list of people you currently follow on Instagram, Pinterest, or other social media platforms. Is their content in line with your recovery process and the shifts you want to make in how you think about your own body? I encourage you to unfollow anyone who posts content that is detrimental to your recovery, and search for more inspiring and self-accepting figures. To practice self-acceptance, create a Pinterest board or collect pictures from magazines and newspapers of bodies that are similar to your *current* body shape. Doing this exercise will help you notice people in a different way, and hopefully allow you to see similarities—rather than differences—between yourself and others.

Confronting Urges

This may be one of the most difficult parts of your recovery: confronting and eventually resisting the urge to binge. In order to do this, you must claim power over the urge. The reasons you shouldn't binge are most likely clear to you, but they haven't helped you stop bingeing. This is because what makes the binge happen is the act of surrendering or abiding the urge. And this urge is coming from a place that does not listen to logic. It comes from the back part of your brain, which is responsible for things like survival and habit behaviors. Yet, your brain has developed the prefrontal cortex in order to use logic and reason to navigate modern day life.

It is important to see the urge for what it is—just an urge. It does not have control or power over you. I will often use the example of when Dorothy meets the "all-powerful Oz" in *The Wizard of Oz*. She thought that he was the only one who could get her back to Kansas, but after lifting the curtain and revealing the truth, she discovers that what she had been searching for externally was actually within her power all along. Your bingeing is not dictated by an all-powerful being, and it isn't something that can be fixed by external rules or guidelines. Your binges are directed by an outdated part of your brain, and it has been reinforced enough to become habitual.

You must pause when the urges arise and allow your inner wisdom to guide you instead.

TAKE ADVANTAGE OF ALTERNATIVE ACTIVITIES

Eventually, your urges will be a fleeting thought, and no alternative action will be necessary to abstain from them. However, in the beginning of your recovery, it is helpful to have a list of activities that you can engage in when you know bingeing tends to occur. This will help you to delay or ideally distract yourself from the urge to binge, and will be beneficial to your overall health and well-being. Even though this means doing more things that you enjoy, there can be a lot of resistance around allowing yourself to do so. You must give yourself permission to do these activities and see them as an investment in your recovery and long-term lifestyle change.

I will often have my clients rate alternative activities from 1 to 10—the higher the number, the more engaging the activity (i.e., 1 = take some deep breaths, 3 = do a house chore or go for a walk, 9 = call a friend).

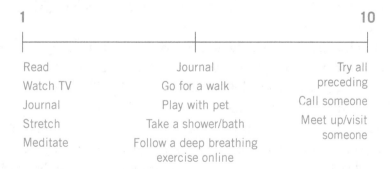

Think back to your last binge. Instead of focusing on the things that led up to the binge, ask yourself at what point you could have stopped mid-binge. Journal about the feelings that are present when asking yourself this question. Does it feel impossible to stop a binge once it's started? If so, visualize what it would be like for you to stop. Imagine yourself putting the food down and walking away. What would you feel as you walk away? What would you feel 10 minutes or 30 minutes after?

"One cannot think well, love well, sleep well, if one has not dined well."
—*Virginia Woolf,* A Room of One's Own

Continued Practice

This chapter addressed how improving the relationship with your body now, in spite of the negativity you may feel toward it, is an essential part of your recovery from binge eating. For a host of reasons, it has become the norm to self-criticize and manipulate our bodies until they become the idealized version associated with beauty and success.

After completing the exercises in this chapter, I hope that you now have a greater connection to your body and see it through a more compassionate lens. Healing your body image will take time, but finding peace with your body is well worth it. In chapter 5, we will explore how you relate to your emotions, their impact on your binge eating, and ways you can embrace them more in order to improve the quality of your life.

CHAPTER FIVE

Managing Your Emotions

Lara, 34, reached out to me after attending a work retreat where she was coached on professional and personal goalsetting. When she was asked about what was holding her back from meeting her goals, it was clear to her that it was her issues with food and her weight. Having this realization spurred her to take action:

> *I am reaching out as I have recently acknowledged how my feelings about my body have taken over my life, and how truly unhealthy and painful it is. Since I was 14, I can't remember a time when I didn't worry about my weight, cancel plans because I felt fat, or analyze my "problem areas" in the mirror each morning. In college, I briefly got down to almost half of my caloric intake and am having fleeting thoughts about trying that again. Even though I know it is not healthy for me and ultimately makes me feel worse, I am lost on how to finally feel good in my body and accept myself.*

When we talked about factors in her life that may have contributed to her body image, Lara revealed that she was definitely impacted by her friends who were also struggling with low self-esteem. But what stood out to her the most were two conversations she had with her parents. When she was 16, she joined a competitive tennis team and began eating more than she was used to, often feeling quite ravenous. She did not like feeling out of control with her food and expressed this to her father. His response was to suggest she try a diet plan, and with a friend, she signed up for Weight Watchers. Thus began her in-depth education of calories and points, and the purchase of her first scale. In college, she gained the "freshman 15" and, while home during winter break, her mom pulled her aside and asked if she thought she had a weight problem. That spurred the drastic cut in her calorie intake and deep insecurity around her body image. Lara believed that neither of the actions by her parents were intentionally mean, and that they would feel terrible if they knew the impact it made on her life.

In order to help Lara free herself of the deep-seated negative body image and diet mentality, we looked more closely at the conversations with her parents and what made those times in her life stand out. When she had the talk with her dad, she was acclimating to joining a new competitive athletic team. She recalled having a lot of anxiety around proving herself to her teammates and pressure to excel. Further, the change in her practice schedule, from twice a week to daily, most likely caused the ravenous hunger cues, as she was expending more energy than she had before joining the new team. Instead of understanding that the increase in hunger was her body's way of keeping her energy levels balanced, or that her feelings were appropriate to the new experience and would not last forever, she jumped to fixing the "problem" by dieting.

Later, when she was asked by her mother about her weight gain, it caused a spiral of insecurity and body shame, fueling even stricter diet rules. As we reflected on how significant of a change she had gone through at that time—moving away from her home, family, and friends to go to college—she was able to be more compassionate with herself. Furthermore, she recognized that, in addition to those changes, her routines, mealtimes, and food options were completely different, and she reflected on how that must have been difficult on her body. She realized that focusing on her weight was an easier way to deal with the deeper emotions she was feeling at the time.

Lara acknowledged that she rarely gives herself time to think about her emotions or how they connect to her body, and she is reluctant to go to friends or family for support. You may relate to Lara's disconnection from the true causes of her emotions. We are rarely given any education on how to understand, acknowledge, and address our emotions in a healthy way. And, even when we do express our feelings, they may be dismissed or disregarded, or we may be judged as being too emotional, sensitive, or needy.

Your Relationship with Your Feelings

Food is woven into our emotional experiences. As hard as you might try, separating the two is impossible. By increasing your curiosity about and reverence of your feelings, you'll be able to make this relationship a positive and beneficial one. Again, if you struggle with binge eating, it does not mean you have tons of emotional baggage you must work through, yet I do think it's safe to assume that your binge eating is currently causing you emotional distress. Just like with other responsibilities we wish we could ignore—credit card bills or the funny noise your car has been making lately—if you avoid it, it will only get worse. And avoiding emotional problems doesn't actually block the anxiety they cause; instead, that anxiety just keeps building like a dark cloud in your periphery.

As you expand your comprehension of the function of emotions, you will be able to use them to your advantage. Unquestionably, there will be times when you will need to compartmentalize or put

YOUR EMOTIONS AND BINGE EATING: HOW ARE THEY RELATED?

Binge eating may have a lot or very little to do with your emotions. Your problem with food does not automatically indicate that you have a problem with your emotions. If you're sure that your binge eating is strongly influenced by your emotions, or if you have experienced a traumatic event that you have not yet healed from, understanding how to manage your emotions will serve you immensely. This does not mean that you must completely heal all of your emotional issues before you can end your binge eating. By and large, the treatment plans I formulate for clients focus on ending the eating disorder behaviors first, and then addressing any emotional issues that lurk under the surface. Of course, there is some emotional education and work being done in conjunction, but we are focused more on what is going on in the present versus the past.

For some clients, once they stopped bingeing, their feelings of anxiety ended, or they felt that they were well enough to do any further emotional work on their own, in a support group, or at a later time. For others, it was important to address the emotions that had been covered up by the eating disorder in order to maintain their recovery. Either way, their quality and engagement in life significantly improved. I hope knowing this further inspires you to remain dedicated to your own recovery and believe in the fact that ending your binge eating is very much attainable.

emotions aside momentarily; this is true for even the most emotionally aware. Your brain and body require breaks from time to time to refuel—not just physically, but emotionally as well. When you allow yourself the time to stop doing or thinking, and relax or take pause in a conscious way, you can refill your emotional tank. By doing so, you enable yourself to address the feelings from a more grounded, calm perspective.

THE DIFFERENCE BETWEEN EMOTIONAL OVEREATING AND BINGE EATING

The desire to turn to food for distraction or comfort is something many people experience. What makes someone an emotional eater versus a binge eater? Emotional eating is when a person eats out of non-physical hunger for a number of reasons. It could mean that they finish the entire bucket of popcorn at the movie theater because they just can't watch a movie without it. Or they get excited at the Thanksgiving dessert table and sample all the pies. In either scenario, the person may experience some discomfort or guilt about eating more than what they were hungry for, but the negative feelings usually end there.

Binge eating is when a person overeats in reaction to being on a restrictive diet or having a restrictive mind-set (i.e., "If I eat desserts I will become fat"). Unlike emotional eaters, instead of guilt, they will feel shame about their eating. When someone feels guilt, he or she feels bad or regretful for something he or she *did*: i.e., "I can't believe I finished that plate of cookies." When someone feels shame, he or she feels like a bad person: i.e., "I can't believe I finished that plate of cookies; I am a worthless human being." Shame is largely connected to a person's senses of self-esteem and self-worth. Someone with an eating disorder believes their self-worth is tied to their ability to control their food and body. Does this feel true to you? If so, in what ways?

PERMISSION TO EMOTIONALLY EAT

As stated in chapter 4, ending the restrictive dieting mind-set is the most influential step to ending a person's binge eating. Yet, once a person stops binge eating, they will still engage in emotional eating. It is important to understand that this is not disordered eating. If you are eating intuitively and no longer follow any food rules or restrictions, then giving yourself permission to emotionally eat is okay.

This may sound counterintuitive or even quite frustrating. After doing the hard work to recover from binge eating, you expect that the desire to overeat will end. However, I have yet to know anyone who does not emotionally eat from time to time. It only becomes a problem when it happens very frequently and is followed by an intense drive to lose weight. For example, when a disordered eater experiences weight gain that they believe is the result of emotional eating, it will spur them to take action to control the symptom (weight gain) rather than the actual problem (feelings that are triggering the frequent overeating). This throws them into the diet cycle, followed by even more self-criticism, disappointment, and hopelessness.

In this chapter, you will learn how to become more aware and accepting of your emotions and how they relate to your bingeing, and discover healthier ways to manage them.

Your Range of Emotions

Emotions often get a bad rap. There are numerous derogatory terms used to describe someone who expresses their emotions: cry baby, wimp, and fragile, to name a few. A common fear is that if you allow yourself to feel your feelings, it will disrupt your ability to get through the day or may cause even greater conflict within a relationship. More often, it is the negative emotions—stress, sadness, and loneliness—that precede the urge to binge eat. But even positive feelings can bring about mindless eating, such as celebrating an accomplishment with a special dessert . . . but then eating the whole cake.

Being aware of your emotions prior to, during, and after binge-ing is extremely helpful in determining what feelings need to be addressed in order to decrease the urge to binge. I know, this is eas-ier said than done. And, most likely, you don't want to think more about the feelings that come up around a binge, especially afterward. But just like with the other tools you have learned thus far, this pro-cess will take patience, curiosity, and self-compassion. As it becomes more obvious to you what you are feeling and needing in the moment, you will be in a stronger position to deny the urge to binge.

When we take a closer look at the timeline leading up to binge behaviors, clients often first respond that it "just happens." They start each day with the best of intentions, but as the day goes on, poor habits or triggers arise and they feel powerless to the urges. Breaking down the moments in minutes or hours just prior to the binge can be helpful in identifying what emotions were present or being ignored. Common patterns to note are the time of day (morning versus evening), the environment (home versus work), part of the week (weekday versus weekend), and the people around you. Noting these patterns will help you understand why there may be more emotional stress or fatigue present, which can then make it much more difficult to stave off a binge. This insight can also shed light on when you *are* able to avoid binges and when you are feeling most attuned to yourself. Focusing on these posi-tive moments will provide information on what is already working for you, and will empower you to build trust with yourself.

HAPPINESS

The pursuit of happiness can lead us to accomplish great things in our lives. Yet, the constant drive to achieve can lead us to endless disappointment, pain, and regret. We often ignore or take for granted the good in our lives because we think things could always be better. The desire for absolute control impedes our ability to shift our expectations or perspectives in ways that could actually lead us to greater happiness. Even when we do acknowledge our happiness, it may be overshadowed by a cloud of unease, as we fear the happiness will go away.

Happiness can very easily become associated with certain foods, and is intertwined with the pleasurable experience of eating. Food and mealtimes tend to be predominant ways we celebrate people and events. For example, after passing an important test, you treat yourself to an all-you-can-eat restaurant or fancy steak house. This is not inherently disordered, but overeating and drinking in the name of celebration can be a slippery slope. If it results in a binge, it diminishes or cancels out the initial happy feelings and replaces them with physical pain and a return to feelings of deficiency.

SADNESS

No one is immune to feeling sad, yet it is rarely talked about or considered appropriate to share unless you've suffered through a major event, such as the death of a loved one. Outside of those circumstances, we are usually encouraged to "just get over it," or are given advice that offers a quick-fix solution. Both of these responses can leave us feeling even more misunderstood and isolated.

Food can provide the non-judgmental comfort we are looking for in those moments. For instance, Jason, 42, had made significant progress in his BED recovery and was rarely experiencing urges to binge. In our most recent session, he shared how his yearly review with his boss went very badly. After learning that he would not be receiving a promotion, he left the meeting shocked and upset, and decided to go to the nearby drive-thru restaurant in order to binge. When he got there, however, he no longer felt the desire to order several things off the menu, and instead ordered a sandwich and fries. He expressed that, although a part of him was proud that he did not binge, he was uncomfortable with having to sit with the negative feelings around the poor review. He missed how the binges would soothe and distract him in those moments. I explained that it is completely normal to grieve the loss of one's binge reflex, and how it will gradually lessen as he continues his work around understanding his emotions.

ANGER

In my formal assessment with clients, I ask them questions about their life history and what brought them to therapy. I also specifically ask how they would describe their relationship to anger. The responses tend to be, "I don't get angry," or "I'm not comfortable with anger." Their answers often give me a good sense as to how they relate to their emotions, and further, how their relationships to food may be outlets for unexpressed anger. When anger is ignored or avoided, it will manifest in other forms—typically in a harmful way against oneself. Not all inklings of anger must be expressed, but becoming more comfortable with the feeling and sensations of it will help you determine the best course of action to take in addressing it.

When this emotion overlaps with our food, the rebellious teenager part of our interior dialogue can take over with great gusto, leading us to make decisions we normally would not make. This part of you is fine with paying the price later on in order to have fun *now*. Another common way displaced anger shows up is when a person feels scrutinized or pressured by someone who wants to "help" them lose weight. They dismiss or even judge their feelings of anger because they believe or tell themselves the person's intentions are altruistic. That may very well be the case, but the negative feelings are real and will be expressed in some way. In many instances, it can lead to a "screw you"-induced binge.

FEELING "FAT"

Even though this is not exactly an emotion, I want to address it here because it is very frequently used by my clients to describe how they are feeling. Often, it indicates a sensation of discomfort in their body and feeling that they are "too much." When clients state they are feeling fat, I ask them to describe the feeling a bit more. In doing so, they are able to reflect on what is actually causing the uncomfortable feeling and redirect their focus to the underlying problem. I also explore with them how long "feeling fat" has been in their emotional dictionaries, and whether there have been times in their lives when they didn't identify or experience this feeling. After some consideration, they will recall particularly happy times in their lives when they felt inspired in their work or by an authentic connection to others. When I ask them what their weight was like in these happier times, my clients are often surprised to remember that they weren't necessarily thinner.

For someone who has never experienced being at or close to their ideal weight, the belief that getting to that number will set them free from feeling fat or uncomfortable in their body is quite impenetrable. One of the ways I attempt to poke holes in this theory is by sharing the fact that *all* of my clients who have an eating disorder (including anorexia) struggle with feeling fat. This feeling does not go away when you reach your goal weight. The feeling will dissipate only when your worthiness is no longer tied to your weight; when reaching that certain number on the scale no longer holds power over you.

DEALING WITH ANGER

Anger is a powerful emotion. Most likely, the last time you felt completely free to express your anger was as a child or infant. Those who consistently ignore the smaller embers of anger may eventually experience the fury of a blaze that only reinforces the fear of anger as an uncontrollable and unnecessary emotion. As a result, people will typically choose to respond to others in whichever way will keep the peace or not rock the boat. Alternatively, they may become rigid and stuck in the anger, acting out of self-righteousness in order to prove the other person wrong. Anger can be a strong conduit for personal change and growth—pushing one to recognize what they are and are not comfortable with. Learning how to experience anger without immediately attaching old thought patterns or reactions will help you use this emotion as another guidepost toward living a more authentic and balanced life.

Nonviolent communication (NVC) is a tool that was designed to specifically improve the way we communicate our feelings of anger to others. This approach delineates the way we express ourselves as violent, such as bullying, blaming, and judging, or nonviolent, using compassion and speech in an authentic manner. The NVC approach values words for their ability to express our needs and understand the needs of others. Lastly, it focuses on *sharing* power with others versus *using* power over others.

> *"Anger is our friend. Not a nice friend. Not a gentle friend. But a very, very loyal friend. It will always tell us when we have been betrayed."*
> —Julia Cameron, The Artist's Way

According to The Center for Nonviolent Communication, "Through the practice of NVC, we can learn to clarify what we are observing, what emotions we are feeling, what values we want to live by, and what we want to ask of ourselves and others. We will no longer need to use the language of blame, judgment, or domination. We can experience the deep pleasure of contributing to each other's well being."

The two parts of the NVC model are:

1. **Empathetically Listening:** Allowing the other person to talk while listening with intention, curiosity, and compassion. This enables you to have a greater understanding of their needs as well as your own.

2. **Honestly Expressing:** Communicating your thoughts and feelings in an honest way in order to get your needs met.

The four components within each part of NVC include:

- Observations
- Feelings
- Needs
- Requests

A common way these components are modeled in couples' therapy is the use of "I" statements. This concept, developed in the 1960s by Thomas Gordon, contrasts "I" statements and "you" statements. While "you" statements tend to express blame to the listener, "I" statements tend to express the speaker's feelings and observations. The use of "I" statements helps to decrease defensiveness and bring about a more honest way of expressing needs and requests. For example, if a couple is arguing about a lack of quality time together, a healthy way to express this would be to say, "I feel neglected and unimportant when you choose to stay out late with colleagues instead of coming home. I would like more quality time together and ask that we plan nights just for us each week."

Write out a list of emotions, aiming for at least 20. If you have trouble, do a quick search on the web for "feelings charts." Once you have the emotions written down, begin to put them in the following categories: "My Most Common/Frequent Emotions," "My Most Difficult/Uncomfortable Emotions," and "The Emotions I Resist/Ignore the Most."

Grab your journal, and without judgment, write about how easy or difficult this exercise was for you. Did you encounter any hesitation or resistance in completing it? Which life experiences may have influenced the categories you placed each feeling in, and what might be keeping you from facing those same feelings now?

The Impact of Stress

Stress is a major factor in most health issues. Out of fear of feeling lazy or being perceived as such, we over-do, over-plan, and over-schedule ourselves. The result is feeling constantly depleted and exhausted, leaving very little time or energy to do the things we enjoy—just for fun. We move through our lives like zombies, just trying to make it through each day.

However, not all stress is inherently bad. It is a feeling that also results from very important and meaningful experiences, such as the stress of preparing and giving a speech at your best friend's wedding or planning a trip abroad. It can be an indicator that you are stepping out of your comfort zone and trying something new and challenging.

RESPONDING TO STRESS

More often than not, when I ask clients what they currently do to relax or burn off steam, their response is, "I eat." It is the only time in their day that they are able to stop thinking, moving, and doing. Understandably, in spite of wanting to end their binge eating, they fear how they will get this respite without turning to food. Recovery from BED does not mean that food as a comfort will end. Instead, it means that food can be a comfort, when needed, without the brutal backlash. Admittedly, food may help to decrease or numb stress in the moment. But it is more like a temporary Band-Aid that is painfully pulled off soon after it is applied. I ask clients to consider whether binge eating actually helps to relieve life stressors, or if it only relieves the stress of fighting off the urge to binge. The discomfort of sitting through an urge can feel like a wrestling match between you and your eating disorder, especially if the solution—however temporary—is just behind the refrigerator door.

As discussed in chapter 4, it is important to recognize that your emotional triggers may fuel the desire to turn to food as comfort, but in order to end binge eating, it is the *urge* to binge that must be addressed. By engaging the more advanced part of your brain, versus the outdated, survival-based part of your brain, you can talk yourself through the urge and choose another way to address the emotions and resume your day. Undoubtedly, as your binges begin to decrease, so too will your stress.

BURN OUT

If early signs of stress are ignored, it can build to unhealthy levels that take a significant toll on your mind and body. If you don't carve out time to relax, your body is forced to perform constantly. Even for people who do take time off or go on vacation, fully disconnecting from life responsibilities or stressors may seem impossible. Perpetual stress impedes your ability to tune into hunger cues, and over time, it causes your body to dull these cues in order to conserve energy. Research shows that almost every system in the body can be influenced by chronic stress. When chronic stress goes unreleased, it suppresses the body's immune system and ultimately manifests as illness.

According to the Office on Women's Health, chronic fatigue syndrome (CFS) affects about 1 million Americans, and women are two to four times more likely than men to be diagnosed. CFS is diagnosed when a person reports symptoms of fatigue that have no other medical cause. The fatigue may worsen with physical or mental activity, but it does not improve with rest.

Symptoms of CFS may include:

- Fatigue

- Loss of memory or concentration

- Enlarged lymph nodes in your neck or armpits

- Unexplained muscle or joint pain

- Headaches

- Unrefreshing sleep

Possible complications of chronic fatigue syndrome include:

- Depression

- Social isolation

- Lifestyle restrictions

- Increased work absences

Hopefully, reviewing the detrimental effects of ignoring your stress will encourage you to value the ways you currently relax and motivate you to implement new methods of self-care in your daily routine. If making changes feels impossible or you are concerned that you may be suffering from CFS, I recommend you schedule an appointment with your doctor or a mental health clinician.

SETTING BOUNDARIES

For those who often find themselves in a caretaking role, the possibility of taking time for themselves or prioritizing their needs over others can feel like an uphill battle. Yet, beginning to establish boundaries in various areas of your life (family, work, friends), especially in the beginning stages of recovery, will help keep you on track with your goals, decrease stress, and create the space you need to work on your recovery. Those who struggle a great deal with putting their needs before others' may be struggling with codependency. Codependence is defined by Merriam-Webster as a person's "dependence on the needs of or control by another." In the book *Codependent No More*, author Melody Beattie states, "Ever since people first existed, they have been doing all the things we label 'codependent.' They have worried themselves sick about other people . . . They have bent over backward avoiding hurting people's feelings and, in so doing, have hurt themselves. They have been afraid to trust their feelings . . . They have struggled for their rights while other people said they didn't have any. They have worn sackcloth because they didn't believe they deserved silk."

Recognizing that you struggle with codependency in some or several of your relationships can be enlightening or disheartening. In either case, acknowledging that taking time for yourself is critical for your well-being, and thus for those you care about, will help you break out of the dynamics that are not serving you and that, most likely, are contributing to the binge eating.

EXERCISE Stress-Reduction Meditation

A tool I share with clients to aid in stress reduction is a loving kindness meditation. It is a Buddhist prayer, and its primary intention is to wish peace and happiness to ourselves, those close to us, and those who surround us but whom we do not know. It also addresses feelings of anger and fosters forgiveness in ourselves and others. You can read through the script on the next page or listen to a version of it online.

Repeating this prayer will help you decrease stress and tension in your body, stay attuned to your feelings, and release what is no longer serving you.

Begin by sitting comfortably. Leave your legs straight out in front of you, uncrossed. You may find it helpful to have one or both of your hands over your heart. As you say each line, allow any feelings that come up to just be, and continue to repeat the words. It may be helpful for you to have an image of someone specific in your mind as well.

My heart fills with loving kindness. I love myself. May I be happy. May I be well. May I be peaceful. May I be free.

May all beings on planet Earth be happy. May they be well. May they be peaceful. May they be free.

May my parents be happy. May they be well. May they be peaceful. May they be free.

May all my friends be happy. May they be well. May they be peaceful. May they be free.

May all my enemies be happy. May they be well. May they be peaceful. May they be free.

If I have hurt anyone, knowingly or unknowingly in thought, word, or deed, I ask for their forgiveness.

If anyone has hurt me, knowingly or unknowingly in thought, word, or deed, I extend my forgiveness.

May all beings everywhere, whether near or far, whether known to me or unknown, be happy. May they be well. May they be peaceful. May they be free.

You Are Not Your Thoughts

We have many, many thoughts throughout the day. Some are unique to the moment and others have been around for years. They can be uplifting or have the power to diminish our sense of self and create the urge to binge or engage in other damaging behaviors. In chapter 2, you learned how CBT uses several thought-changing tools to help shift unwanted behaviors. It can often feel overwhelming or simply impossible to stop the thoughts that do not serve you. Instead, you can direct your focus on distancing yourself from them to reduce their impact.

ACKNOWLEDGING NEGATIVE THOUGHTS

Many of the fear-based thoughts that run through your mind are in response to a core belief you hold about yourself—for example, that you are unlovable or unintelligent. These beliefs inform how you see yourself, others, and your life experiences. As Anais Nin writes in *Seduction of the Minotaur*, "We don't see things as they are, we see things as we are." Core beliefs are rigid, usually formed during childhood, and always on the hunt for any evidence to prove their validity. As a result, a great deal of your recovery work will be behind the scenes—acknowledging the thoughts in your mind and recognizing which ones tend to lead you down paths you no longer want to go down.

Earlier in this book, you also learned that your brain is wired to retain negative memories and thoughts more vividly than positive ones as a way of survival. You were also encouraged to name or compartmentalize the parts of you that try to proffer these negative memories and thoughts as facts.

Another technique in line with the acceptance and commitment therapy (ACT) approach to disempower negative thoughts is to literally try to visualize the words in your mind. See the words spelled out, in quotes, or as an advertisement on a billboard. Can you notice the thoughts and, instead of pulling over to correct what is written on the billboard, just keep driving past it? You are still aware of them, but with practice, you can skip determining whether they are valid and instead continue on without getting pulled into negative behavior patterns or habits. Additionally, you might try to imagine someone (perhaps a celebrity or a person in government) who you do not respect saying the negative commentary to you. When you hear the thoughts in this way, it may make it easier to disregard or laugh them off. Adding some humor to this process doesn't hurt and can quickly facilitate a shift toward a more fair, positive state of mind.

Lastly, when you believe a situation cannot change, your brain's ability to think outside the box or consider different ways of doing something diminishes. Can you recall a time when you really wanted to do or buy something, did not have the means, yet *somehow* you found a way to make it happen? Phrases like "the stars aligned" or "it fell into my lap" may be used to explain it, but most likely your thoughts in relation to what you wanted contributed toward achieving it.

"What progress, you ask, have I made?
I have begun to be a friend to myself."
—Hecato

EXERCISE   Thought Tracking

One way to track and create the space for altering your thoughts is to keep a small notebook with you at all times, use an app, or keep a document on your phone or laptop. Taking a few moments to observe your thoughts and emotions throughout the day allows you to address them in the moment and challenge automatic negative thoughts. After a binge, feelings such as intense shame, sadness, and regret may be present. Sitting with these emotions may lead to even further destructive behaviors, such as bingeing again or deciding to "get back on track tomorrow morning" in an attempt to compensate for the binge. By tracking these thoughts, you can integrate more empowering self-talk, such as, "I need to move on from this, tomorrow is a new day" or, "I deserve more support and will focus on more self-care tomorrow."

Additionally, maintaining a regular eating schedule is key to resetting your body's hunger and satiety signals. The starvation or restriction pattern is a common trap ultimately resulting in a binge. Noting the urge to punish yourself or turn to past coping methods will help you to recognize and end these patterns.

"If you hear a voice within you say, 'you cannot paint,'
then by all means paint and that voice will be silenced."
—Vincent Van Gogh

Self-Care and Self-Love

Throughout the chapters thus far, I have used the term *self-care* when discussing substituting eating disorder behaviors with activities that are soothing, comforting, or enjoyable. This may feel superfluous to the hard work of ending your binge eating, but from my experience, the most dramatic shifts happen when clients take this part of their recovery seriously. Creating space in your day to get out of your head and do something that calms your nervous system or fulfills your soul is like a direct affront to the eating disorder.

REMEMBER YOUR VALUES

Connecting self-care activities to your values will help you prioritize these activities as necessary components on the journey toward a more authentic identity or version of yourself. I think it's safe to presume that a value of yours is to improve your relationship with those you love. By spending time with them in ways that are truly engaging, such as going for a hike in nature or playing tennis or a board game, you can bridge these two values. In many ways, self-care tends to overlap with our values. For example, traveling may be a value for you. Seeing it as an excellent form of self-care adds to the worthwhileness of the time and investment you put into planning it.

EXERCISE Journal Activity

Reflect on which parts of this chapter were specifically hard for you and which parts were inspiring or new. In what ways would you like to hold yourself accountable to practicing the tools you learned in your life this week? Is there anyone you would like to share them with?

Continued Practice

In this chapter, you expanded your emotional vocabulary and learned constructive ways to deal with your emotions without repressing them. Further, you learned about the ability of emotions to help you make decisions, voice your needs, and set boundaries that are aligned with your goals and values. The differences between emotional eating and binge eating were explained, and we looked at the impact that stress has on both. Lastly, we addressed how to connect to your anger and communicate it in a way that is authentic and respectful to both parties in a conflict.

In the final chapter, you will be given recommendations on how to integrate the tools you have learned into your life. Most importantly, the next chapter will foster the mind-set that a balanced and happy life is best obtained by looking internally, not focusing on changing external factors.

CHAPTER SIX

Start Living

In a recent session with my client Alma, she hesitantly shared with me her decision to go on a certain popular diet because several of her family members and boyfriend were doing it in order to lose weight for her sister's upcoming wedding. Her sister, who was the first to go on the diet, went on about how great she was feeling in her body and all the weight she had lost. I could hear the excitement and hope in Alma's voice as she talked about how she was enjoying planning meals, grocery shopping, and cooking according to the diet guidelines with her boyfriend.

As her therapist, I did my best to bring compassion to her decision. I understood that in spite of some great things occurring in her life recently—graduating from her master's program, moving in with her boyfriend, and being offered a highly competitive internship—she was feeling overwhelmed by all of the changes and was in search of something that felt concrete and within her control. She had been doing so well in her recovery work that we reduced our sessions to once a month. But as she continued to share about her life over the last few weeks, she disclosed that she had binged and purged (vomited) the previous weekend. She had been alone the entire weekend, and her mood was quite low. She tried to do some self-care activities (yoga class, watch movies) to help shift her mood, but they only seemed to bring her down even more. She experienced a strong urge for her favorite snack, Pringles chips, and allowed herself to have them, even though they were not an acceptable food according to the diet's rules. She expressed feeling extremely guilty for eating the chips and ashamed that she purged, since the last time she had done that was almost a year ago.

In our work together, she had been able to move this snack out of the "forbidden food" category and allowed herself to have it when she wanted it. Yet, because it was swiftly relegated back into that category per the diet's guidelines, it triggered her shame around failure and lack of willpower, feelings made even worse because it seemed like her boyfriend was able to follow the diet so easily. I encouraged her to be gentle with herself around the underlying need for more control and structure in her life. I reviewed with her how, in spite of any weight loss, her body will fight to return to its initial weight. I also pointed out how she could use some of the things she did enjoy from the diet for any number of non-diet recipes, such as preparing her grocery list ahead of time and cooking more with her boyfriend. Further, she could use this experience as motivation to deepen her recovery.

> *"It is easier to prevent bad habits than to break them."*
> *—Benjamin Franklin*

Navigating Different Meal Settings

Each meal provides its own set of obstacles. But thinking it through and preparing ahead of time is the best way to stay in tune with your hunger cues and avoid the urge to binge. Some creative, out-of-the-box thinking will be helpful, as your weekday and week-end routines are likely different, and meals you make at home will differ from those you have at a family member's house. One of the many great things about intuitive eating is that it considers our desire to socialize, which often entails eating. Being an intuitive eater does not preclude you from any activities, but preparing ahead of time (for any and all meal environments) will enable you to honor your hunger cues more accurately and in a more timely manner.

PLANNING AHEAD

Creating a meal plan or schedule is beneficial in a variety of ways. Doing so may satisfy your need for structure, and it can decrease the time spent on assessing the cabinets and/or fridge for what to make. This is also financially beneficial, as you can have meals prepared that will keep you from spending money on restaurants, ordering in, or making multiple trips to the grocery store. Even if you don't feel like cooking for the week, you can still prepare a list of meals that are easy for you to pick up on your way home from work or that are simple to prepare at home. When going to a restaurant, it may be helpful to look up their menu online and get a sense of what you might like to have, or read reviews of popular dishes to help inform your decision.

CREATING A SNACK PACK

Many of my clients keep snack packs on-hand at all times to avoid becoming too hungry in between meals or when they find themselves in a situation where they do not like what is available. One client became sold on the idea after having a terrible flight experience. Due to a weather delay, she was stuck on the tarmac for two hours without any food available before a three-hour flight. She thought she would be fine, having eaten her lunch prior to boarding. But halfway through her flight, her hunger returned, soon followed by headaches and extreme agitation. Since then, she carries a small tote in her bag that includes some dried fruit, string cheese, nuts, and a small bag of popcorn or chips. Again, this will take some prudence in planning ahead and keeping the pack stored in your desk, car, or bag, but it can be extremely beneficial to curbing impulsive meal choices, feeling unsatisfied with whatever is available, or becoming ravenous.

MAKING ADJUSTMENTS

In order to spend time with others, attend events, and answer your body's needs for fuel, you may need to make some adjustments to your typical meal schedule. In the initial phase of transitioning to intuitive eating, you are strongly encouraged to keep as much of a regular eating schedule as possible (eating every three to four hours) in order to retrain your body to know and trust that it will consistently be fed and refueled.

For instance, a client and I worked out how he could navigate his meal schedule around an evening networking event. He knew there would be some snacks available at the event, but most likely not enough to substantiate a meal. We decided that his best bet was to eat his dinner early to avoid becoming too hungry and possibly triggering an urge to binge. What if, instead of eating prior to the event, he waited until after? Most likely, he would have been quite hungry and would be more inclined to pick up a quick and easy meal to satisfy his high level of hunger. He then would likely eat very quickly and have a larger portion than usual, leaving him feeling uncomfortably full. It is important to expect these scenarios, ride out the feeling of fullness (usually around 20 minutes), and trust your body will recalibrate as necessary.

EXERCISE   Meal Planning

Now that you've seen the benefit of planning out your meals, write a plan for the next day, several days, or week. Consider the structure of your day and designate preferred meal times. Once you have those blocked out, think about what meals you would like to have at each of those times. Remember, this plan can be as flexible as you would like, so choose the foods that you think you might enjoy. By creating a master list of your favorite meals for breakfast, lunch, dinner, dessert, and snacks, you can simplify this process even more. As you go through your meal schedule, you can easily go through the master list and plug in your meals.

Flexibility is key to intuitive eating, so including an alternate option or two allows you to make a more intuitive decision in the moment. For example, while meal planning for the week, you may recall that on Wednesday you have a meeting at noon and will need to eat lunch later than usual. So, you might decide to plan on a more robust breakfast option for that day and include a morning snack in order to sustain you until lunch. Additionally, consider what meals are easiest to prepare, and save those for nights when you know you won't have much energy to cook.

As for the format of your meal plan, choose one that will be the most accessible to you, so you can easily reference it throughout your day. Some options include:

- A small notepad you can carry with you

- Your phone (notes app or calendar)

- A recovery app (Recovery Record and Rise Up + Recover are great ones)

- An Excel or Google Docs spreadsheet

- An activity chart you can download and print

At the end of your day or week, reflect on how your meals went and how closely you were able to follow your plan. Remind yourself that this is not about counting calories or judging the food. Note what positive things happened as a result of the meal plan. About what percentage of it were you able to follow? What got in the way (practical issues or disordered eating thoughts), and is there anything that should be adjusted or changed? This is not about perfection or succeeding or failing; you are working toward having a greater understanding of your body's needs and investing effort into having a more balanced life.

Mindful Shopping

It's understandable if you feel lost and overwhelmed in a grocery store. Shelves stocked full of a vast variety of foods can easily throw anyone off their intended course. Learning how to make this process more comfortable and even enjoyable will further add to the ease in which you plan, cook, and savor your meals.

DON'T SHOP HUNGRY

A common trigger is shopping when hungry. Depending on your level of hunger, your ability to be attuned to your body's needs may be drowned out by feelings of weakness, agitation, or intense hunger. Instead, eat a meal before you go shopping to avoid impulse purchases. Understandably, shopping soon after eating may not always be possible, nor can you always know when you will be hungry. Having your snack pack with you (in a purse/tote/suitcase/pocket/car) will help you with unexpected hunger. If you feel yourself starting to get hungry while shopping, give yourself permission to end the shopping trip early.

STOCKING FOOD

Nutrition experts have differing opinions on how much food a person should stock in their home. Ideally, you should store enough food to offer a variety of meals with little waste. Yet, when healing disordered eating, the decision around what type and how much food to keep in your kitchen is multilayered. For example, Ben (from chapter 4) did not keep bread in his home because it had become a trigger food for him. Instead of continuing to try to avoid or cut out bread (which was clearly not working), he agreed to keep it in his home. By facing the fear, he eventually was able to have bread around without triggering a binge.

My hope for you is that you will end all power struggles with food and will be able to keep any type of food in your home without fear of bingeing. My recommendation to clients is to keep a substantial supply of their fear foods at home. For example, if chips were on your forbidden foods list, you should keep four medium bags stocked at all times. As you allow yourself to eat the foods that you have eaten only infrequently or during binges, your brain will no longer register them as something new and exciting. Just like with leftovers, after a few days you will tire of the food and desire something else. Having an ample supply will suppress the rebellious voice that says, "This is your last chance to have this!"

By keeping trigger foods stocked, you are training your mind and body to learn that:

1   These foods are no longer restricted as part of a diet or restrictive mind-set.

2   You have full permission to eat whatever you are craving.

3   There is no longer a reason to fear or compensate for the feeling of scarcity.

4   Occasional emotional overeating is okay.

I understand that this may feel like a setup to binge. And yes, binges might occur. But, clearly, keeping these foods out of your house or in very small portions has not kept you from bingeing, either. No matter how much you control the food in your house, you cannot control the food or your cravings for it outside of your house. If you are ready to bring an end to the tug-of-war with food, let go of the rope. The thoughts and urges to binge will decrease as you engage with them less and less and begin to trust yourself more and more.

EXERCISE   List Making

Another way to improve your grocery shopping experience is to bring a prepared shopping list. Having a list will help you remember all the items you need and keep you from browsing aimlessly, inevitably being distracted by items you did not intend to buy. Below are some key components to a robust list; use this as a framework for your own.

❏ Produce   ❏ Snacks

❏ Meat/seafood   ❏ Bread

❏ Frozen foods   ❏ Pasta/rice

❏ Canned goods   ❏ Condiments

❏ Cereals/breakfast foods   ❏ Beverage

❏ Dairy/cheese/eggs

"It's a beautiful thing to have lungs that allow you to breathe air and legs that allow you to climb mountains, and it's a shame that sometimes we don't realize that that's enough."
—Unknown

Movement Plan

Just as you're working toward creating more balance and variety with food, so too can you create this relationship with movement and exercise. Between obsessive/daily and resistant/non-existent,

IMPROVING YOUR GROCERY SHOPPING EXPERIENCE

In addition to planning ahead, here are a few more things you can do to help make grocery shopping feel like less of a stressful chore:

- Try different stores to find the one you feel most comfortable in (even if it is farther from home/work).
- Plan out the time you want to spend there—i.e., from 3 p.m. to 3:45 p.m.
- If possible, go during a weekday to avoid crowds.
- Ask a friend, roommate, significant other, or family member to go with you.
- Wear headphones and listen to your favorite music while you shop.
- Make plans for something fun or relaxing afterward.

If grocery shopping is just not something you enjoy, accept your feelings around it and consider other options. You could ask a friend, roommate, significant other, or family member to go for you or add the items you need to their next trip. Additionally, many grocery stores offer online delivery or pick-up services. Lastly, another way to diversify your meals and add to your cooking skills is to try one of the many online companies that send you meal kits with instructions and all the ingredients you need to cook delicious meals.

where do you fall on the exercise spectrum? How did this pattern develop for you, and have there been times when it was different? The amount and way you exercise is significantly influenced by the relationship you have with your body. If you consider your body something that cannot be trusted and must be controlled, you will choose activities that are not enjoyable and are fused with punitive rules and judgments. If your relationship with your body is one of avoidance, so too will be your feelings around engaging in any mindful movement or exercise.

Most likely, your current approach to exercise will need to shift in order to foster greater balance and sustainability. For someone with BED, the typical mentality is to use exercise as a way to compensate for overeating or bingeing. By integrating more positive movement in your life, you can slowly break down this mind-set. Exercise for fun or to benefit mental and physical health has been shown to be a much better motivating force than the goal of weight loss.

When you feel ready to address this part of your recovery, consider the forms of exercise you would like to do, and how and when you will do it. In what ways can you incorporate movement into your daily routine? Blocking time out in your calendar and exercising at a regular time each day or week will help you avoid conflict and keep you motivated. But just like with intuitive eating, you must allow yourself to decide in the moment if your body truly needs exercise. Give yourself permission to rest if it feels like that is what your body actually needs. Overall, remember that this is meant to be a form of self-care that helps reduce stress. If it feels like focusing on movement at this time is increasing stress, give yourself permission to take a break or put it aside for now. When you're ready, you can reevaluate the why, how, when, and what.

If your weight is a significant factor that you feel prohibits you from trying new forms of movement, know that decreasing sedentary habits alone can make a significant impact on your health. This is true for anyone at any size, regardless of the amount of exercise they engage in. Just becoming more aware of the length of time you sit and reminding yourself to stand, walk around, or stretch after an hour of sitting will bring significant improvements to your health. Any way that you are able to add more movement to your life is a success in self-care if it is done from a self-loving place and not as a form of punishment or compensation. Below is a brief list of activities to consider.

- Intramural teams (volleyball, basketball, soccer, kick-ball, bowling)

- Weight lifting, cross training, or other gym activities (take advantage of a day pass or free trial to see if you feel comfortable)

- Classes such as Zumba, yoga, or boxing

- Guided online exercise videos

- Golf

- Martial arts

- Rock climbing

- Running/jogging

- Skiing/snowboarding

- Swimming

- Tennis

In addition to or instead of those activities, some suggestions for increasing your movement routine include:

- Park farther away from the store or your work.

- Play with or take your dog for a walk.

- Take the stairs versus the elevator.

- Go for a walk during lunch.

- Use a standing desk at work.

  Ways to make exercise more enjoyable and intentional:

- Play outside with your children.

- Work with a personal trainer (make sure their approach aligns with yours!).

- Listen to a podcast.

- Make a playlist of your favorite energizing songs.

- Ask a supportive person to join you.

- Buy new exercise clothing and shoes.

- Remind yourself of the last time you enjoyed exercise and how good you felt during and after.

- Engage in positive body image affirming activities (i.e., positive body talk in front of the mirror, acknowledge gratitude for your body).

EXERCISE Your Scale

For my clients, the scale is a tool to track their weight, but it rarely provides the reassurance or motivation they seek. Each time they step on the scale, the critical voice is right there with them. Due to the slightest increase in weight, their day is ruined as they spiral down into self-criticism and shame. It also reignites the quick-fix appeal of diets. Even if the number on the scale is down, your critical voice will jump in and demand you keep up the work. By and large, my advice to clients is to get rid of their scales. Stopping or at least decreasing the use of your scale will help you establish a more considerate relationship with your body. Refocusing the intention from weight-control to improving your behaviors with food is the only path to freedom.

For this exercise, decide if you will be getting rid of, putting away, or decreasing the use of your scale. Take out your journal and write about your relationship to the scale. How it has helped you and hurt you? What are you hoping will change as a result of the action you chose to take? If you decided not to alter your use of it at all, what are your reasons why?

Adding Professional Support to Your Recovery Plan

If you're considering or are curious about working with someone to support you on this journey toward intuitive eating, I encourage you to pursue the options that are available to you. When you work one-on-one with a clinician or health coach, you are supported each step of the way. They will not only help you stay on track toward recovery, but they will also most likely help you accelerate the process.

When researching professionals to help you treat your disordered eating, make sure to get a clear understanding of their philosophies and approaches to treating BED. Many providers may also share their own personal stories of recovery, and most approaches will typically involve some CBT, ACT, and mindfulness skills along with meal planning. Many of my clients benefited from a more structured approach at the beginning, and then gradually transitioned to intuitive eating toward the conclusion of our work together. Treatment options and trained professionals to help with BED include:

- **Nutritionist/Registered Dietitian (RD):** Professionals with this title have completed a bachelor's degree in dietetics, food science, or nutrition and may also have a master's degree in similar specialties. RDs will support you by creating an individualized plan around food and movement that will foster your ability to nourish your body and become more attuned to your hunger cues. They are also able to support you in healing while navigating certain allergies or medical conditions. Dietitians often work in tandem with a mental health clinician and medical doctor when treating someone with an eating disorder.

- **Licensed Mental Health Clinician:** At minimum, these providers hold master's degrees in counseling, psychology, or social work. For those who specialize in treating eating disorders, they most likely received training through providing individual, family, and group counseling in a treatment program facility. Your work together will address your current life concerns and how your childhood or past experiences impact the changes you would like to make.

- **Health Coach:** Their focus is on creating an individualized plan for you to achieve health and wellness. They may use worksheets or other interactive tools to help you integrate these changes.

- **Support Groups:** Healing your disordered eating among peers who are also struggling may strengthen your resolve and motivation to recover. There are a variety of group formats, from drop-in style (like a 12-step or community group) to closed groups where a strict commitment is required. If you are considering a 12-step group, I suggest looking for Overeaters Anonymous (OA) or Eating Disorders Anonymous (EDA) meetings in your area and staying away from Food Addicts (FA), as they require following rigid food guidelines.

- **Residential, Partial Hospitalization, or Intensive Outpatient Program (RTC/PHP/IOP):** If you believe that your disordered eating is at a place where your life is being extremely compromised by the obsessive thoughts and behaviors, taking time off from work or school to commit to a treatment program will help you accelerate your healing and provide you the space to give it your full attention. Treatment typically includes meeting with a medical doctor, therapist, and dietitian in addition to group therapy and meal support.

Getting Help from Friends and Family

Another critical component to sustaining your progress is receiving support from others. The people in our lives, from friends and family to colleagues or classmates, impact us in a variety of ways. Choosing to share more details about your life and recovery may bring up painful feelings of anxiety and vulnerability. Yet the overall benefits of welcoming supportive people into your life far exceed any negative feelings that may come from opening up to them in moments of struggle.

In a talk at TEDx Houston, Brené Brown stated, "Owning our story can be hard, but not nearly as difficult as spending our lives running from it. Embracing our vulnerabilities is risky, but not nearly as dangerous as giving up on love and belonging and joy—the experiences that make us the most vulnerable. Only when we are brave enough to explore the darkness will we discover the infinite power of our light." Trust in this process of peeling back the layers of your story, and acquiesce to them all, both the good and the bad, as they make up who you are. As you do this, you will feel the freedom of true self-acceptance.

A possible first step to sharing your story would be to call an eating disorder hotline or join an online forum for recovery (see Resources, page 139). Any step that you take out of isolation, secrecy, and shame will bring you closer to your recovery.

MAKE YOUR INTENTIONS KNOWN

As you decide who you want to include in your recovery journey, consider the level of detail you feel comfortable disclosing and what type of support you need from the people with whom you choose to share. Understandably, you hope that whomever you choose will be compassionate, understanding, and perhaps even express a genuine interest in joining you on this path toward self-acceptance and freedom with food. Ideally, they would quickly understand and support you 100 percent. Unfortunately, that may not be the outcome or response you receive. Depending on their own relationship with food, this can be a very loaded topic for some people, eliciting a wide variety of opinions and "facts." Patience will be key as you navigate the ways others respond to the changes you make as a result of your new mind-set. Change is typically afflictive to the person going through it, but it can also create unease in those close to them. They may respond and act in ways that surprise or disappoint you. By working on maintaining an open dialogue, you can address feelings in the moment or swiftly quell others' concerns or perceived judgments. Accept that you may need to clearly state and restate your goals and intentions. Doing this not only helps them understand, but it also affirms the goals and intentions for you as well.

WHEN PEOPLE DON'T UNDERSTAND

Your body is YOUR body. This path is about bringing you back to a place where you are able to understand its unique needs for nourishment, movement, pleasure, and rest. The eating disorder has led you away from this internal power, leaving you even more susceptible to marketing ploys and others' opinions.

I recently had a phone session with Angela, a client who sought my support about two years ago for her eating disorder. I no longer see her on a regular basis, as she made significant progress in her recovery, healing her seven-year struggle with restriction, over-exercising, and binge eating. During our work together, she addressed not only the binge behaviors but also the areas in her life that were making her unhappy. Four months ago, she decided to quit her job and pursue her dream of living abroad in order to become fluent in Spanish (as well as have some amazing experiences). In our check-in session, she shared how she struggled with second-guessing her decision, especially now that her parents and friends began to question her more and more about her return date. Angela didn't *feel* ready to return, but also wondered if some of her family's concerns were valid. I asked if she could remember a time when she did not agree with or understand a decision that one of her siblings had made regarding their own health or well-being. She recalled how her brother had complained of feeling very low and "off," leading her and her family to presume his low energy was a result of mild depression. He felt adamant that the cause was physical, not solely an emotional issue. He went to several doctors for consultations and blood tests. Eventually, he was diagnosed with Lyme disease. Luckily, he trusted himself enough to know something was not right in his body and persevered in spite of a great deal of naysaying and dissent.

Seeing how her concerns about her brother may have been quite logical—yet ultimately incorrect—helped Angela let go of some resentment she was feeling toward her own naysayers and regain more trust within herself.

SCRIPT FOR TALKING TO FRIENDS AND FAMILY

Knowing how to respond to the people closest to you can be tricky to say the least. I have heard countless stories of the pain that remains long after the act of bullying or "harmless" critiques are made.

I have no doubt that you have your own stories around the insensitivity and ignorance of others. Learning how to navigate these situations will help you respond in whatever way feels right and respectful to you and your process. Below are some common questions you may be asked and some suggestions as to how you can respond.

Q: Why can't you just stop [insert eating disorder behavior]?

A: Healing from an eating disorder is a bit more complicated than that. Trust me, I wish it were that easy! For a variety of reasons, the way that a lot of people turn to food for comfort or a distraction became more intense for me. It is tough work to recover, but I feel like I am on the right path. I appreciate your patience in this, as it does take time.

Q: This diet worked for me, why don't you try it?

A: Thanks, but I'm not into diets anymore. They've never really worked for me, and after doing some research, I have actually learned that only 5 percent of people succeed at losing weight and keeping it off for more than five years.

Q: You look different/great, have you lost weight?

A: I actually don't (or am trying not to) pay attention to my weight that much anymore. I've found the less I think about it, the better I feel.

Q: What do you mean you're not dieting anymore? Don't you want to lose weight/feel good/be healthy?

A: I definitely want to be healthy and feel good, but I've come to the realization that focusing on losing weight has actually kept me from those things. I take my health very seriously, but I no longer want to be a slave to the scale. Instead, I'm going to make more of an effort to listen to my body's needs. I want to enjoy my life more, not suffer through it waiting for the number on the scale to validate it.

Q: I don't get how intuitive eating works. Can you explain it to me?

A: I appreciate you wanting to understand intuitive eating. It took some time for me to wrap my mind around the approach as well, but after reading the principles, it made a lot of sense to me. To eat intuitively basically means to follow your own hunger cues as a guide to decide when, what, and how much to eat, instead of following a diet. If you'd like to learn more, I encourage you to do your own research. Whether you agree with it or not, I hope you will respect my decision, as I believe it is the right one for me.

Q: How can I help in your recovery? Do you want me to tell you when I think you're overeating?

A: Thank you for wanting to support me in this journey. A lot of it will have to be done on my own (or with the support of a profes-sional), and I prefer that you not turn into the food police. That will most likely make me feel more uncomfortable and anxious during our meals together. Instead, just checking in with me in general about my day or how I am feeling will help me get out of my head and into the present moment.

In general, try to be as clear as possible with those closest to you about what you would like and not like said about your food, appearance, or exercise. My clients will usually tell loved ones that they do not want to feel like they are being watched or questioned about their food. You can let them know that it's okay if they don't "get it" or know what to say or do, as you are both learning as you go. They can do their own research, consult with a professional, or read books on the topic of healing eating disorders (like this one) in order to improve their level of understanding. This will be tremendously beneficial to your relationship and your recovery. Additionally, increasing quality time together and respecting the time you both take for your own self-care will ease any tension that might arise. Ultimately, though, the responses and actions of others are not in your control, and your recovery cannot be dependent on them. This is about you and your process.

Continued Practice

I hope that you now feel prepared with the insight and tools needed to continue your journey. Within each chapter, I included many of my clients' stories in an effort to decrease feelings of isolation or hopelessness that have kept you from committing to recovery in the past. Just like what you may be experiencing at this juncture, they struggled with the fear that they were not capable or even deserving of recovery. Yet, with each step they took, however cautiously, they proved that fear wrong.

*"Our greatest glory is not in never falling,
but in rising every time we fall."*
—Oliver Goldsmith

One Day at a Time

As you continue taking steps toward mindful and intuitive eating, you will inevitably run into some roadblocks. You may become frustrated with yourself when, in an attempt to diversify your meals, you order something new at a restaurant that you end up extremely disliking. Or, in an attempt to make sure you are following the principles of intuitive eating correctly, you might feel like a failure each time you feel uncomfortably full. Yet, in order to make consistent progress in your recovery, failure must be a copacetic part of the process. If not, it will contort intuitive eating into just another diet—one where you "fail" with the slightest error. The degree that a person fears failure typically correlates to their level of perfectionism. For those who possess high levels of perfectionism, their tunnel vision–like outlook on life leads them to unreasonably high expectations that, when cannot be met, send them down a spiral of self-loathing, blame, and regret.

As you read this book, did it seem like your self-critical voice became louder in certain chapters versus others? If you skipped some or all of the preceding exercises, do you think perfectionism was a factor in the decision? Self-talk such as "If I can't do it right, I may as well not do it at all" is a common attitude that keeps us from taking steps toward change. Other common thoughts that cover up the fear of failure are, "I'll get to it later" and "I have more important things to do." In order to become more comfortable with failure, you must be able to forgive yourself, let go, and move on. As you practice this, you will become better at setting more reasonable expectations for yourself, thus decreasing the amount of negative self-talk that paralyzes you.

Remember: what we resist persists. Even after making significant cognitive and behavioral changes, you will continue to face moments where you would rather ignore or give in to overwhelming feelings or urges. As in any other worthwhile pursuit, you will inevitably face challenges. I hope that you listen to the part of you that is calling out for something different. Every time you listen to that part, you are closer to making peace with food. Apply the steadfastness you brought to the diets to your recovery. When you become aware that you may be depriving yourself of something, consider the reasons why. This deprivation of food or life experiences leads to neediness, and when needs go unanswered, some form of comfort is desired. Thus far, that search for comfort has resulted in binge eating. As you move forward in your recovery, instead of engaging in a power struggle with food, *you* will be in charge. If you feel in charge of your decisions, you will no longer feel that bingeing just happens to you.

I hope that no matter where you go from here, you consider the impact your decisions around food and exercise have on your mental health and overall quality of life. I hope that you will no longer compromise these qualities or values solely for your physical health or weight loss. Perhaps, your life will become more about choosing the foods you like to eat, spending time with people you care about, and doing activities that bring you joy and make you feel alive.

Resources

Websites

- About-Face.org
- AntiDietRevolution.org
- BEDAOnline.com
- ChristyHarrison.com
- DanaFalsetti.com
- HAESCommunity.com
- KelseyMiller.com
- LindaBacon.org
- NAMEDInc.org
- RecoveryWarriors.com
- SizeDiversityandHealth.org
- TheBodyPositive.org
- TheMilitantBaker.com
- TheProjectHeal.org

Books

- *Diet Survivor's Handbook: 60 Lessons in Eating, Acceptance and Self-Care*, by Judith Matz, LCSW, and Ellen Frankel, LCSW. Naperville, IL: Sourcebooks, 2006

- *Don't Diet, Live-It! Workbook: Healing Food, Weight & Body Issues*, by Andrea Wachter, LMFT, and Marsea Marcus, LMFT. Carlsbad, CA: Gürze Books, 1999

- *Eating in the Light of the Moon: How Women Can Transform Their Relationship with Food Through Myths, Metaphors, and Storytelling*, by Anita A. Johnston, PhD. Carlsbad, CA: Gürze Books, 1996

- *8 Keys to Recovery from an Eating Disorder: Effective Strategies from Therapeutic Practice and Personal Experience*, by Carolyn Costin and Gwen Schubert Grabb. New York. W.W. Norton & Company, 2012

- *Food and Feelings Workbook: A Full Course Meal on Emotional Health*, by Karen R. Koenig, LCSW, EdM. Carlsbad, CA: Gürze Books, 2007

- *Intuitive Eating: A Revolutionary Program that Works*, by Evelyn Tribole, MS, RD, and Elyse Resch, MS, RD, FADA, CEDRD. New York: St. Martin's Griffin, 2003

- *Intuitive Eating Workbook: Ten Principles for Nourishing a Healthy Relationship with Food*, by Evelyn Tribole, MS, RDN, and Elyse Resch, MS, RDN. Oakland, CA: New Harbinger Publications, Inc., 2017

- *Rules of "Normal" Eating: A Commonsense Approach for Dieters, Overeaters, Undereaters, Emotional Eaters, and Everyone in Between!*, by Karen R. Koenig, LCSW, EdM. Carlsbad, CA: Gürze Books, 2005

- *Secrets of Feeding a Healthy Family: Orchestrating and Enjoying the Family Meal: How to Eat, How to Raise Good Eaters, How to Cook*, by Ellyn Satter, MS, RD, LCSW, BCD. Madison, WI: Kelcy Press, 2008

MINDFULNESS

- *Beyond Dieting: Psychoeducational Interventions for Chronically Obese Women: A Non-Dieting Approach*, by Donna Ciliska, RN, PhD. New York: Brunner/Mazel, Inc, 1990

- *Big Girl: How I Gave Up Dieting and Got a Life*, by Kelsey Miller. New York: Grand Central, 2016

- *Embody: Learning to Love Your Unique Body (and Quiet That Critical Voice!)*, by Connie Sobczak. Carlsbad, CA: Gürze Books, 2014

- *Fat Is Not a Four-Letter Word*, by Charles Roy Schroeder, PhD. Minnetonka, MN: Chronimed Publishing, 1992

- *The Mindfulness and Acceptance Workbook for Anxiety: A Guide to Breaking Free from Anxiety, Phobias, and Worry Using Acceptance and Commitment Therapy*, by John P. Forsyth, PhD, and Georg H. Eifert, PhD. Oakland, CA: New Harbinger Publications, Inc., 2016

- *Things No One Will Tell Fat Girls: A Handbook for Unapologetic Living*, by Jes Baker. Berkeley, CA: Seal Press, 2015

- *200 Ways to Love the Body You Have*, by Marcia Hutchinson, EdD. Berkeley, CA: Crossing Press, 1999

- *When Women Stop Hating Their Bodies: Freeing Yourself from Food and Weight Obsession*, by Jane R. Hirschmann and Carol H. Munter, New York: Ballantine Books, 1996

References

Chapter One

American Psychiatric Association. *Diagnostic and Statistical Manual of Mental Disorders, Fifth Edition*. Washington DC: American Psychiatric Association Publishing, 2016.

Aniston, Jennifer. "For The Record." *Huffington Post*. Accessed August 2018. https://www.huffingtonpost.com/entry/for-the-record_us_57855586e4b03fc3ee4e626f.

Bulik, Cynthia M., and Eliana Perrin. "Obesity and Anorexia: How Can They Coexist?" Association for Size Diversity and Health. Accessed August 2018. www.sizediversityandhealth.org/content.asp?id=34&articleID=216.

Culbert, K.M., S.E. Racine, and K.L. Klump. "Research Review: What We Have Learned about the Causes of Eating Disorders—A Synthesis of Sociocultural, Psychological, and Biological Research." *Journal of Child Psychology and Psychiatry* 56, no. 11 (2015): 1141–64 doi: 10.1111/jcpp.12441.

Davis, Caroline, Robert Levitan, Caroline Reid, Jacqueline Carter, Allan Kaplan, Karen Patte, Nicole King, Claire Curtis, and James Kennedy. "Dopamine for 'Wanting' and Opioids for 'Liking': A Comparison of Obese Adults With and Without Binge Eating." *Obesity* 17, no. 6 (June 2009). doi:10.1038/oby.2009.52.

Eating Disorder Hope. "Eating Disorder Statistics & Research." Accessed August 2018. www.eatingdisorderhope.com/information/statistics-studies.

Hudson, J.I., E. Hiripi, H.G. Pope, Jr., and R.C. Kessler. "The Prevalence and Correlates of Eating Disorders in the National Comorbidity Survey Replication." *Biological Psychiatry* 61, no. 3 (February 1, 2007): 348–58. doi:10.1016/j.biopsych.2006.03.040.

Kassirer, J.P., MD, and M. Angell, MD. "Losing Weight—An Ill-Fated New Year's Resolution," *New England Journal of Medicine* 338 (1998): 52–54. doi: 10.1056/NEJM199801013380109.

Le Grange, D., S.A. Swanson, S.J. Crow, and K.R. Merikangas. "Eating Disorder Not Otherwise Specified Presentation in the US Population." *International Journal of Eating Disorders* 45, no. 5 (July 2012): 711–18. doi:10.1002/eat.22006.

Mann, T., A.J. Tomiyama, E. Westling, A.M. Lew, B. Samuels, and J. Chatman. "Medicare's Search for Effective Obesity Treatments: Diets Are Not the Answer." *American Psychologist*, 62, no. 3 (2007): 220–33. doi: 10.1037/0003-066X.62.3.220.

Mann, Traci, PhD. *Secrets From the Eating Lab: The Science of Weight Loss, the Myth of Willpower, and Why You Should Never Diet Again.* New York: Harper Wave, 2017.

Martin, Crescent B., Kirsten A. Herrick, Neda Sarafrazi, and Cynthia L. Ogden. "Attempts to Lose Weight Among Adults in the United States, 2013–2016." NCHS Data Brief No. 313 (July 2018). National Center for Health Statistics. www.cdc.gov/nchs/products/databriefs/db313.htm.

National Association of Anorexia Nervosa and Associated Disorders. "Eating Disorders Statistics." Accessed August 2018. www.anad.org /education-and-awareness/about-eating-disorders/eating-disorders-statistics.

Schwartz, Barry. *The Paradox of Choice: Why More Is Less.* New York: Ecco, 2016.

Smink, F.E., D. van Hoeken, and H.W. Hoek. "Epidemiology of Eating Disorders: Incidence, Prevalence and Mortality Rates." *Current Psychiatry Reports* 14, no. 4 (August 2012): 406–14. doi:10.1007 /s11920-012-0282-y.

Chapter Two

Brach, Tara, PhD. *Radical Acceptance: Embracing Your Life with the Heat of a Buddha*. New York: Bantam Dell, 2003.

Costin, Carolyn, and Gwen Schubert Grabb. *8 Keys to Recovery from an Eating Disorder: Effective Strategies from Therapeutic Practice and Personal Experience*. New York: W. W. Norton & Company, 2012.

Ikeda, J.P., P. Lyons, F. Schwartzman, and R.A. Mitchell. "Self-Reported Dieting Experiences of Women with Body Mass Indexes of 30 or More." *Journal of the American Dietetic Association* 104, no. 6 (June 2004): 972–4. doi:10.1016/j.jada.2004.03.026.

Kuk, J.L., M. Rotondi, X. Sui, N. Blair, and C.I. Ardern. "Individuals with Obesity But No Other Metabolic Risk Factors Are Not at Significantly Elevated All-Cause Mortality Risk in Men and Women." *Clinical Obesity*, July 12, 2018. doi:10.1111/cob.12263.

Linehan, Marsha, PhD, ABBP. Dialectical Behavior Therapy. https://behavioraltech.org/dialectical-behavior-therapy-dbt.

Miller, Kelsey. *Big Girl: How I Gave Up Dieting and Got a Life*. New York: Grand Central, 2016.

Neff, Kristin, PhD. https://self-compassion.org

Original Intuitive Eating Pros. "10 Principles of Intuitive Eating." Accessed August 2018. http://www.intuitiveeating.org/10-principles -of-intuitive-eating.

Robinson, Eric, Paul Aveyard, Amanda Daley, Kate Jolly, Amanda Lewis, Deborah Lycett, and Suzanne Higgs. "Eating Attentively: A Systematic Review and Meta-Analysis of the Effect of Food Intake Memory and Awareness on Eating." *The American Journal of Clinical Nutrition* 97, no. 4 (April 2013): 728–42. doi:10.3945/ajcn.112.045245.

Salzberg, Sharon. *A Heart as Wide as the World: Stories on the Path to Lovingkindness*. Boston: Shambhala Publications, Inc., 1997. (Page 104)

Schwartz, Jeffrey M. *You Are Not Your Brain: The 4-Step Solution for Changing Bad Habits, Ending Unhealthy Thinking, and Taking Control of Your Life*. New York: The Penguin Group, 2011.

The Center for Mindful Eating. https://thecenterformindfuleating.org.

Tribole, Evelyn, MS, RD, and Elyse Resch, MD, RD, FADA. *Intuitive Eating: A Revolutionary Program that Works*. New York: St. Martin's Griffin, 2003.

Chapter Three

Brown, Brené, PhD., LMSW. *The Gifts of Imperfection: Let Go of Who You Think You're Supposed to Be and Embrace Who You Are.* Center City, MN: Hazelden, 2010.

Costin, Carolyn, and Gwen Schubert Grabb. *8 Keys to Recovery from an Eating Disorder: Effective Strategies from Therapeutic Practice and Personal Experience.* New York: W. W. Norton & Company, 2012.

Fletcher, Anne M., MD, RD. *Sober for Good: New Solutions for Drinking Problems—Advice from Those Who Have Succeeded.* New York: Houghton Mifflin, 2001.

Hanson, Rick. *Buddha's Brain: The Practical Neuroscience of Happiness, Love, and Wisdom.* Oakland, CA: New Harbinger Publications, Inc., 2009.

Kahn, Sheira, MFT, and Nicole Laby, MFT. *Erasing ED Treatment Manual: Tools and Foundations for Eating Disorder Recovery.* Charlston, NC: CreateSpace, 2012. (Page 36)

Oxford Living Dictionaries. "Spirituality." Accessed August 2018. https://en.oxforddictionaries.com/definition/spirituality.

Rock, David, MD, and Daniel J. Siegel, MD. "The Healthy Mind Platter." Accessed August 2018. http://www.drdansiegel.com/resources /healthy_mind_platter.

Tolle, Eckhart. *The Power of Now: A Guide to Spiritual Enlightenment.* Novato, CA: New World Library, 2004.

Chapter Four

Anchor, Shawn. *The Happiness Advantage: The Seven Principles of Positive Psychology that Fuel Success and Performance at Work.* New York: Crown Business, 2010.

Bacon, Linda. *Health at Every Size: The Surprising Truth about Your Weight.* Dallas, TX: BenBella Books, Inc., 2008.

Eating Disorder Hope. "Eating Disorder Statistics & Research." Accessed August 2018. https://www.eatingdisorderhope.com/information/statistics-studies.

Grodstein, F., R. Levine, L. Troy, T. Spencer, G.A. Colditz, and M.J. Stampfer. "Three-Year Follow-Up of Participants in a Commercial Weight Loss Program: Can You Keep it Off?" *Archives of Internal Medicine* 156, no. 12 (June 24, 1996): 1302–6. https://www.ncbi.nlm.nih.gov/pubmed/8651838.

Gustafson-Larson, A.M., and R.D. Terry. "Weight-Related Behaviors and Concerns of Fourth-Grade Children. *Journal of American Dietetic Association* 92, no. 7 (July 1992): 818–22. https://www.ncbi.nlm.nih.gov/pubmed/1624650.

Homan, K.J., and T.L. Tylka. "Appearance-Based Exercise Motivation Moderates the Relationship Between Exercise Frequency and Positive Body Image." *Body Image* 11, no. 12 (March 2014): 101–8. doi:10.1016/j.bodyim.2014.01.003.

Johnston, Anita A., PhD. *Eating in the Light of the Moon: How Women Can Transform Their Relationship with Food Through Myths, Metaphors, and Storytelling.* Carlsbad, CA: Gürze Books, 1996.

Matz, Judith, and Ellen Frankel. *Beyond a Shadow of a Diet: The Therapist's Guide to Treating Compulsive Eating.* New York: Brunner-Routledge, 2004.

National Center on Addiction and Substance Abuse (CASA) at Columbia University. "Food for Thought: Substance Abuse and Eating Disorders." 2003. https://www.centeronaddiction.org/addiction-research /reports/food-thought-substance-abuse-and-eating-disorders.

National Eating Disorders Association. "Statistics & Research on Eating Disorders." Accessed August 2018. https://www.nationaleatingdisorders .org/statistics-research-eating-disorders.

Neumark-Sztainer, Dianne. *"I'm, Like, SO Fat!": Helping Your Teen Make Healthy Choices about Eating and Exercise in a Weight-Obsessed World.* New York: Guilford Press, 2005. (Page 5)

Robison, Jon, Kelly Putnam, and Laura McKibbin. "Health at Every Size®: A Compassionate, Effective Approach for Helping Individuals With Weight-Related Concerns Part I." *American Association of Occupational Health Nurses Journal* 55, no. 4 (April 2007). doi:10.1177 /216507990705500402.

Roth, Geneen. *Women Food God: An Unexpected Path to Almost Everything.* New York: Scribner, 2010.

Shisslak, C.M., M. Crago, and L.S. Estes. "The Spectrum of Eating Disturbances." *International Journal of Eating Disorders* 18, no. 3 (November 1995): 209–19. https://www.ncbi.nlm.nih.gov/pubmed/8556017.

Tovar, Virgie. Description of key note speech entitled "#LoseHateNotWeight." https://www.virgietovar.com/blog /virgie-to-keynote-fat-activism-conference.

Tylka, T.L., and N.L. Wood-Barcalow. "The Body Appreciation Scale-2: Item Refinement and Psychometric Evaluation." *Body Image* 12 (January 2015): 53–67. doi:10.1016/j.bodyim.2014.09.006.

Chapter Five

Beattie, Melody. *Codependent No More: How to Stop Controlling Others and Start Caring for Yourself.* Center City, MN: Hazelden, 1986.

Beck Cognitive Behavior Therapy. "What is Cognitive Behavior Therapy (CBT)?" Accessed August 2018. https://beckinstitute.org/get-informed /what-is-cognitive-therapy.

Cameron, Julia. *The Artist's Way: A Spiritual Path to Higher Creativity, 25th Anniversary Edition.* New York: TarcherPerigee, 2016.

Chödrön, Pema. *When Things Fall Apart: Heart Advice for Difficult Times.* Boulder, CO: Shambhala Publications, Inc., 1997.

Gordon, Thomas, PhD. "Origins of the Gordon Model." Gordon Training International. Accessed August 2018. http://www.gordontraining.com /thomas-gordon/origins-of-the-gordon-model.

Lerner, Harriet, PhD. *The Dance of Anger: A Woman's Guide to Changing the Patterns of Intimate Relationships.* New York: Harper & Row, 1985.

Mayo Clinic. "Chronic Fatigue Syndrome." Accessed August 2018. https://www.mayoclinic.org/diseases-conditions/chronic-fatigue -syndrome/symptoms-causes/syc-20360490.

Merriam-Webster.com Dictionary. "Codependence." Accessed August 2018. https://www.merriam-webster.com/dictionary/codependency

Pearlin, Leonard I., Scott Schieman, Elena M. Fazio, and Stephen C. Meersman. "Stress, Health, and the Life Course: Some Conceptual Perspectives." *Journal of Health and Social Behavior* 46, no. 2 (June 1, 2005): 205–19. doi:10.1177/002214650504600206.

Razali, Salleh Mohd. "Life Event, Stress and Illness." *The Malaysian Journal of Medical Sciences* 15, no. 4 (October 2008): 9–18. https://www.ncbi.nlm.nih.gov/pmc/articles/PMC3341916/#.

The Buddhist Centre. "Loving-Kindness Meditation." Retrieved August 2018. https://thebuddhistcentre.com/text/loving-kindness-meditation.

The Center for Nonviolent Communication. "The 2 Parts and 4 Components of NVC." Accessed August 2018. http://www.cnvc.org/Training/the-nvc-model.

The Office on Women's Health. "Chronic Fatigue Syndrome." Accessed August 2018. https://www.womenshealth.gov/a-z-topics/chronic-fatigue-syndrome.

Chapter Six

Bosomworth, N.J. "The Downside of Weight Loss: Realistic Intervention in Body-Weight Trajectory." Canadian Family Physician 58, no. 5 (May 2012): 517–23. https://www.ncbi.nlm.nih.gov/pubmed/22586192.

Brown, Brené. "The Power of Vulnerability." TEDxHouston. https://www.ted.com/talks/brene_brown_on_vulnerability/up-next.

Centers for Disease Control and Prevention. "Physical Activity and Health." Accessed August 2018. https://www.cdc.gov/physicalactivity/basics/pa-health/index.htm.

Owen, Neville, Genevieve N. Healy, Charles E. Matthews, and David W. Dunstan. "Too Much Sitting: The Population-Health Science of Sedentary Behavior." *Exercise and Sport Sciences Reviews* 38, no. 3 (July 2010): 105–13. doi:10.1097/JES.0b013e3181e373a2.

Tylka, T.L., R.A. Annunziato, D. Burgard, D. Danielsdottir, E. Shuman, C. Davis, and R.M. Calogero. "The Weight-Inclusive versus Weight-Normative Approach to Health: Evaluating the Evidence for Prioritizing Well-Being over Weight Loss." *Journal of Obesity* 2014. doi:10.1155/2014/983495.

Voss, Michelle W., Timothy B. Weng, Agnieszka Z. Burzynska, Chelsea N. Wong, Gillian E. Cooke, Rachel Clark, Jason Fanning, Elizabeth Awick, Neha P. Gothe, Erin A. Olson, Edward McAuley, and Arthur F. Kramer. "Fitness, but Not Physical Activity, Is Related to Functional Integrity of Brain Networks Associated with Aging." *NueroImage* 131 (May 1, 2016): 113–25. doi:10.1016/j.neuroimage.2015.10.044.

Index

Acknowledgments

Writing this book has truly been a dream come true. Thank you to Callisto Media and my editor Nana K. Twumasi for supporting me in bringing my approach to healing to those who are in search of a life free of binge eating.

Heartfelt appreciation to Roya Bahrami, Laura Fraser, Rochelle Greenhagen, Ana Mazdyasni, Sara Aslan, Catherine Mevs, and Robert Thomas—your generosity of time, insight, and encouragement during the writing of this book (and beyond) means more than you know.

To my Evolve Wellness team: Anna Clark, Lauren Korshak, Natalie Makardish, Nicole Klawitter, Kari Floberg, Erika Bent, Sarah Calloway, Jennifer Simmons, and Cora Keene, thank you for believing in my vision of providing outstanding holistic treatment to those struggling with eating disorders. I feel honored to work alongside such a dedicated, compassionate, and talented group of women. I am indebted to Christine Pappas for bringing me into the field of eating disorder treatment and showing me the way. And to Nova Goldberg, thank you for listening.

I am deeply grateful to my family and friends, near and far, for your love and support, especially Raquel Bahrami-Baalbaki, Nasrein Bahrami, and Mina Bahrami.

Lastly, Reza, Maysan, and Zahra, thank you for inspiring me to play, dance, and laugh more and for being my greatest sources of joy.

About the Author

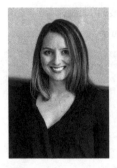 **SHREIN H. BAHRAMI** is a licensed therapist in San Francisco. She is the founder of Evolve Wellness, a group practice of clinicians specializing in the treatment of eating disorders. For nearly a decade, she has provided counseling in residential and outpatient settings to clients and their families seeking recovery from anorexia, bulimia, and binge eating disorder. Shrein has contributed to articles featured on NBC News, *The Guardian*, Bustle, *Reader's Digest*, Romper, and The Mighty. Learn more at www.shreinbahrami.com.